The Mothers' Book

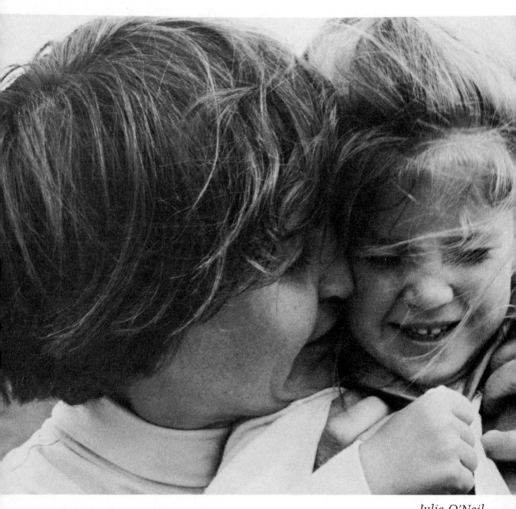

Julie O'Neil

The Mothers' Book

SHARED EXPERIENCES

Edited by Ronnie Friedland and Carol Kort

Houghton Mifflin Company   Boston   1981

Grateful acknowledgment is made to the following for permission to reprint material copyrighted or controlled by them:

"Birth/Caesarean" copyright © 1981 by Carol Hoffman DeCanio. Used by permission of the author.

"Plague" by Kinereth Gensler, copyright © 1976 by Kinereth Gensler. From *Three Some Poems* by J. Dobbs, K. Gensler, and E. Knies (Alice James Books). Reprinted by permission of the author.

"The Meeting Is Imminent" by Carol Kort. First published in *Sojourner.* Copyright © 1978 by Carol Kort. Reprinted by permission of *Sojourner* and the author.

"The Children" by Susan MacDonald, from *Ms.* magazine, July 1972. Copyright © 1972 by Ms. Magazine Corporation. Reprinted by permission of *Ms.* magazine and the author.

"Night Feeding" by Muriel Rukeyser, from *Selected Poems* 1951. Copyright © 1968 by Muriel Rukeyser. Reprinted by permission of Monica McCall, International Creative Management.

Library of Congress Cataloging in Publication Data

Main entry under title:

The Mothers' book.

 1. Mothers — United States — Addresses, essays, lectures. 2. Mother and child — Addresses, essays, lectures. 3. Mothers — United States — Psychology. I. Friedland, Ronnie. II. Kort, Carol.
HQ759.M89   306.8'7   80-24938
ISBN 0-395-30527-6
ISBN 0-395-31134-9 pbk.

Printed in the United States of America

P 10 9 8 7 6 5 4 3 2 1

We dedicate this book to Joshua and Eleza,
quite literally our inspiration.

Acknowledgments

First and foremost, we would like to express our gratitude to Bette Rothman, whose creative mind came up with the original idea for this book.

We are also extremely indebted to Bonnie Burt for all the time and energy she spent collecting the photographs for the book, as well as for her advice as a photographer and as a friend.

For offering their time, advice, and support, we would also like to thank Simone Bloom, Paul Friedland, Patricia A. Moore, William Novak, Lisa Weil, and all the participants from the Mothertalk group.

American Baby magazine deserves special mention for running a notice which enabled us to reach mothers of all kinds, from all over the country. We also appreciate the editorial assistance provided by Frances Tenenbaum at Houghton Mifflin, and the understanding provided by the staff members of the Special Programs Office at the Harvard Graduate School of Design.

To our husbands, Dan and Michael, thank you for your ideas, encouragement, and help — particularly all the extra child care — from the beginning to the end of our project.

Last, our gratitude to all the mothers and friends who contributed in some form, taking out time that they did not have, and supporting and advising us in our venture. Without them and their network, this book would not have been possible.

Contents

15. Foster, Adoptive, and Natural Mothers

16. Teenage Mothers

17. Feelings About Surgical Deliveries

18. Mothering Children with Special Needs

19. When Things Go Wrong

20. Dealing with Death

21. Dealing with the Future

Introduction

This book was conceived out of our recognition that the transition to motherhood changes a woman's life abruptly and totally, and that knowing how other mothers cope with their feelings during these changes could provide necessary support and guidance. As mothers ourselves we had observed that new mothers need some idea of what to expect, as well as emotional support for what they are feeling. Presenting the whole range of emotional responses mothers have to pregnancy, the postpartum period, working, staying at home, and altered relationships with husbands, mothers, friends, and selves would, we hoped, respond to this need.

Our own experiences as mothers differed greatly. One of us endured a terrible pregnancy and birth, while the other breezed through both. One of us loved the first six months of motherhood, while the other suffered through a painfully long postpartum period. One of us consciously chose not to work while raising a young child and is still nursing her two-year-old, while the other returned to work when her infant was a half-year-old and stopped nursing after a year. Each of us felt terribly alone and lost during her own difficult periods and wondered if anyone else had had similar experiences. Reading about another mother's trying pregnancy or postpartum adjustment would have helped us better understand and cope with our own.

As we sat planning this book over coffee, after our infants had finally been tucked in their cribs for the night, we set as our goal the task of conveying what it *feels* like to be a mother today. How does it feel not to nurse when today's climate is so unabashedly pro-nursing? How does it feel to have a negative reaction to your child when you first see him or her? How does it feel to have no sexual interest in your husband for months after the birth of your child? How does it feel to relate to your own mother once you have become a mother? How does it feel to institutionalize a retarded child? How does it feel to be an unmarried or a lesbian mother?

We went to the source to learn about motherhood — from the mothers themselves. We set out to reach mothers from every part of the country, mothers of all ages and kinds — single mothers, stepmothers, mothers who adopted, mothers of children with special needs, and mothers who had lost a child. We contacted both working and stay-at-home mothers who had something to share, whether it was ambivalence, doubt, guilt, or joy. We reached mothers who stay home with pleasure and those who feel that they must. Our book includes personal accounts by very traditional mothers and by ardent feminists. We asked a group of mothers to talk freely about sexuality and motherhood; we asked a mother from Texas to write about nursing her adopted child; we asked teenage mothers to share their feelings of isolation. We wrote to mothers who live in beach towns and big towns, in Utah and in Illinois, on the East Coast in suburbia and on the West Coast in San Francisco.

Although we have included mothers of all ages, many of our contributors are in their early or mid-thirties, part of a recent trend for women to become mothers later in life. These older mothers often expressed satisfaction that they had explored other sides of themselves before becoming mothers.

The messages we received from mothers clearly dispelled the Supermom and Superwoman myths. Rarely is motherhood "naturally" easy. More often parents feel ambivalence. Countless women wrote to us about loving yet sometimes hating their child; loving their child but hating the demands of motherhood; and loving their child but finding themselves too exhausted, depleted, and overwhelmed to express this love.

We learned what it feels like to have a child with Down's syndrome or cerebral palsy, to have a child who dies. We learned about anger, jealousy, and shame. We heard from a mother who was frustrated by her gifted child, a mother who had battled infertility, a mother whose infant has cancer. We learned that more and more mothers are having Caesarean sections and that the shock of unplanned surgery and its aftermath, while adjusting to new motherhood, is often difficult to cope with. And we heard mothers' anguish and sorrow in the face of larger world forces, unable to protect their children.

We feel we have provided a forum for mothers undergoing

emotional transitions of all kinds to speak about themselves and their issues honestly. With all its highs and lows, our book is a positive affirmation of motherhood. We wish that a book such as ours had been available when we were considering motherhood, and when we became mothers.

In motherhood,
Carol Kort and Ronnie Friedland
Brookline, Massachusetts, and Cazenovia, New York
June 1980

1

Pregnancy

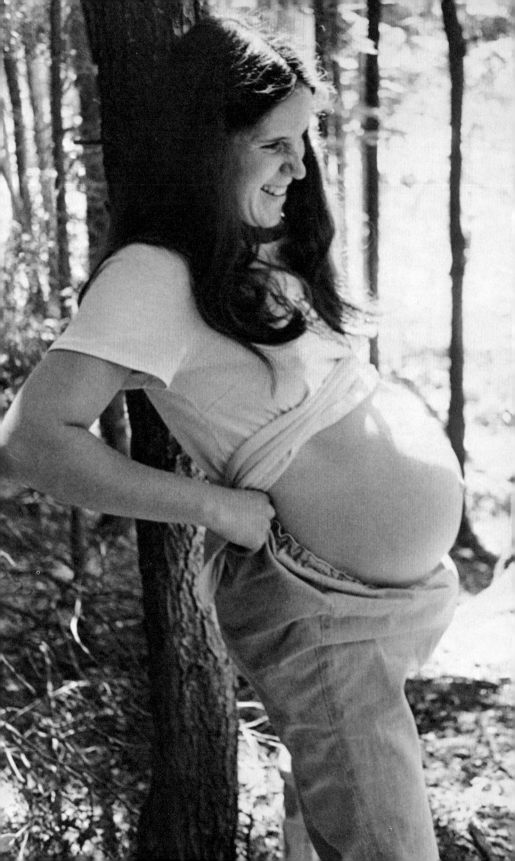

The Meeting Is Imminent

CAROL KORT

Four Months Pregnant
This morning I heard my child speak in a heartbeat.
It filled the sterile room, warmed the cold stirrups.
I heard it as a pounding of an elephant herd.
I was filled with its urgency, its unabashed rhyme.

Beat, little tiger, beat on in my ballooned womb.
Let your life song be heard; already you are strong.
Pump furiously, little heartbeat, pump to your own time.
This morning I heard my child speak her first word.

Six Months Pregnant
I have disappeared. I taste like a prune pit.
Where is my pulse, a crazed night, a sudden flush?
I am filled with child, blood of another.
I have emptied all else to be that being's mother.
Give me back my madness, an unplanned touch.
I am a frozen cervix. I want back my other.

Eight Months Pregnant
The meeting is imminent.
I am breathless. You crush me.
Breathless too as waiting for a lover
who comes certainly, but at a time unappointed.
My tough little fruit pit, for comfort
will you prefer the womb to the breast?

My skin is taut. You churn in the drum.
Feet kick daringly through the stretched canvas.
I can almost touch the toes
through the bloated belly with its meandering veins.
The meeting is imminent.

3

You are more real than anyone in my life.
But you are not real.
I carry you everywhere in my gut.
But you are not here.
I am your mother/giver/maker.
Tremendous is my body and my love for you.
Soon the fruit blossoms into flower.
The meeting is imminent.

Four Weeks Old
I am growing my daughter this summer, thrush and all.
Marigolds pale against her golden aura.
Her eyes are snapdragon saucers,
her thighs are dimpled jade plants — rubbery and thick.
She smells of milkwood and daisies.
She clings like a vine but wanders like the Jew.
Her heart-shaped lips are delicate as pussy willow.
Everything about her turns upward — buttercups to light.
This burgeoning bouquet was rooted in my womb.
Next summer I will again plant nasturtium and pansies.
This summer I am growing my daughter, a flower
   extraordinaire.
Her beauty will drive you mad, but she must not be picked.

Metamorphosis of a Pregnancy

GINNIE KUHN MITCHELL

It was one of those close-friend moments, several of us standing
around in the kitchen, wrapping up dinner dishes and conversation.

4

We were warm from the wine and still-radiating oven. Suddenly I became sick. I was as amazed as everyone else, but the puzzling wave of nausea passed as quickly as it had come, and I soon felt fine. In our wine-warm silliness, we started speculating that it must be the food, the booze, a bug going around, or pregnancy. The last suggestion brought a slew of wisecracks because of the weight I had put on that month. No, I rationalized, it was the Christmas cookies in which I had freely indulged.

It was on an annual business trip to Florida that I was again forced to face the possibility of pregnancy. My pants would not close, even after weeks of post-Christmas dieting. I had to wear a loose dress the whole time. One evening, a mother of two looked long and hard at me, and declared that my belly contained a baby. "No, no," I countered. I told her about the Christmas cookies and explained that Mark and I were not yet ready for children. She smiled; I didn't.

Later that night, lying wide awake in a hot, stale motel room, something moved in my belly. A small sort of roll, but enough to make me think, What on earth was that? It dawned on me, and I was no longer disbelieving. I sobbed in shock and fear, and in anger that I had repudiated what had been happening to my body the past four months.

During the twelve-hour drive home from Florida, I thought of names for the baby. Mark, my husband, was still disbelieving, refusing to play my "game." In the silence between Adam and Adrienne, I began to sense how terribly difficult it would be for him to accept this pregnancy. I thought about all our conversations about waiting to have children until we were more settled, ready and able to cope with all that having children entailed. We had always agreed, but we had never discussed or even considered the possibility of an accidental pregnancy. Until now. And Mark still wasn't willing to discuss it.

When we got home I made an appointment to see the doctor. I was feeling moments of pure joy alternating with moments of terrible indecision. All the way to the appointment, Mark reminded me of our prior decision to wait and of our commitment to our newly established business and to each other as a twosome. He was very serious, and I became very frightened. I had believed that when

5

it really came down to it, he too would be delighted to be expecting a baby. But here he was telling me that he would rather not have one.

―――――――

I had enough time sitting on the examining table, cold and vulnerable in my stiff paper shift, to work myself into a state of anxiety as I waited for the results of the urine test. My doctor breezed in, white-coated and intoning the obligatory "How are you today, Mrs. Mitchell?" while simultaneously reading my chart. "Congratulations," he said, "it looks like you are going to be a mother. Let's slide all the way down here, that's right, and see just how far along you are."

It was a relief to know that I had been right, but now I had to *deal* with it. I wanted to scream. Instead, I cried. Once I explained the dilemma, the nightmarish scene dissolved, and the uncaring ogre became a kind, sympathetic Marcus Welby ally. He asked if I would consider an abortion, no simple procedure at a confirmed four months. I thought for a moment and knew that I could not live with myself if I took that course.

―――――――

Mark was very quiet all the way to our lunch date, and the next hour was spent talking business.

Later, still silent, Mark retreated to the bedroom, staring into his thoughts. I tried unsuccessfully to coax him out of it, and then stormed into the living room cursing fate, diaphragms, and our rotten potency. We moved through the next few days in silence so heavy it hurt. I felt let down, sad, and very lonely.

A few days later, while we were watching television, I felt what could only be the baby kicking. "Quick!" I cried to Mark. "Put your hand here." And right on cue the baby kicked again, hard and unmistakably. We looked at each other and wept. We wept not in self-pity, but in awe at what we had inadvertently created. And we wept in joy. This was our baby, not an untimely swelling of my womb. This was a life, a child, our child.

―――――――

There were bad days when I was not quite big enough for the world to know I was pregnant rather than fat. And there were days when I was so tired that I could not move, when my emotional cup ran over, and I thought that I would drown.

There were bad nights too. I had trouble sleeping, and my anxieties grew larger as the hour grew later. I was afraid and I felt guilty for being afraid. I feared the pain, the responsibilities, the way this baby would alter our lives. I feared the unknown. I am no longer a child, I thought in the night. I am the mommy now. I will never again be the child. A little voice deep within me cried, You're not ready. It's diapers and feedings and becoming a haggard housewife from now on, kid. And at two in the morning I believed that voice and cried myself to sleep. I had been such a staunch defender of the positive aspects of having a child that I didn't dare wake Mark and let him see my fear, ambivalence, and weakness.

Reading proved my ally and salvation. I read everything I could get my hands on about pregnancy and childbirth. I started asking questions, ate well, and exercised daily. Gradually I began to love my ever-expanding belly. We were a team, two against all. I became stronger each day as I became more aware of and more comfortable with what was going on within me, and by my third trimester I had finally and fully accepted the pregnancy.

Mark had slowly grown stronger also, more confident and much more excited about the prospect of having a baby. As the birth approached, he proved himself to be all I could ask for in terms of a wonderful husband and father-to-be. In fact, Mark and I became incredibly close. I still found myself crying, but now because I felt the child in my womb to be so dear to us.

In my ninth month, I would sit in the nursery, windows open, mild breezes wafting new curtains, aware of the fragrance of sweet spring and the almost-summer sunshine. The warm yellow sun made the bright nursery colors even brighter, and the room was soft and glowing, like a newborn itself. I, too, was spring, ready to bloom. I'd sit in the wicker rocker, secondhand and repainted, looking around the room at all things in readiness for our baby. Everything was little, neat, sweet. There was the afghan that kept my belly warm while I made it, the shower gifts from loving friends, and the wicker bassinet from my mother, which had been mine as

7

an infant. After having denied the reality of pregnancy so vehemently, here I sat, holding my belly, overwhelmed with love.

After spending thirty months at home with her daughter, GINNIE KUHN MITCHELL is preparing to open up a clothing store in a small beach town on the southeastern coast of North Carolina.

Mothertalk

A GROUP DISCUSSION ON PROBLEMS WITH PREGNANCY

CANDY: One of the happiest moments of my life was when I found out I was pregnant.

RACHEL: I was also ecstatic when I found out I was pregnant, and so was my husband. But we were both totally unprepared for what my pregnancy was like. I soon began feeling nauseated twenty-four hours a day. It felt like I had a bad stomach flu that never went away.

SARAH: It was constant nausea for me also. Every day by the time I got to work I would be so ill that I would have to lie down. The nausea was horrible, depressing, and shocking: I never had expected pregnancy to be that way. I kept wondering, Why me?

RACHEL: In addition to feeling sick, I could barely get up in the morning because of the fatigue. I would be up for an hour, then sleep for hours, then be up for an hour again. I simply could not keep myself awake. I began to question whether I would ever again be myself. I feared that for the rest of my life I would be this mindless blob, unable to read or to do anything I normally enjoyed.

CANDY: I never realized how lucky I was to have had a great pregnancy. It sounds so frightening, Rachel.

RACHEL: It was. The situation was even worse because we had moved recently to a new city where I didn't know anyone. So I had no support. There was no one there who knew what I *used* to be like.

SARAH: I felt like something was taking over my body, and I was angry about it. I had expected to feel connected to this child in a wonderful, spiritual way. But more and more I had a sense that I was being invaded by this being whose needs always came first and were often in conflict with my own.

CANDY: Can you give an example of what you mean?

SARAH: Yes. I didn't feel like eating at all because of the nausea, but I forced myself to eat well so the fetus would develop properly. I began to be afraid that since pregnancy was such a disappointment, motherhood would be also. Fortunately, it wasn't, and I adore my child.

BETH: My experience was exactly the opposite of yours. Because I had a difficult time getting pregnant in the first place, I was delighted when I became pregnant. I literally had no pregnancy symptoms: I didn't have sore breasts, I wasn't sick, I wasn't tired. I felt absolutely normal. But I was petrified that I was going to have a miscarriage, because I had read that a typical pregnancy that ends in a miscarriage is one with no pregnancy symptoms. So I panicked because I *didn't* feel pregnant.

CANDY: I just had a typically good pregnancy — very few physical or mental problems at all. But let's get back to Sarah. What happened after the first four months?

SARAH: The fatigue went away. I had two good months. Then it was summer, and I had three really rotten months: I was very uncomfortable, waddled about, and felt continual discomfort from the heat. And I had thought that you were supposed to feel great all the time!

CANDY: You certainly must not have felt sexual at all.

SARAH: That was the least of my concerns. My major goal during pregnancy was to get through each day, and to hope that it would get better the next day. I could never think far ahead enough to envision the baby, or how I would feel as a mother. I became swallowed up in the present.

BETH: That was your first pregnancy. What about this one — now that you're in your ninth month?

9

SARAH: The second time around it has been much harder because I have to take care of my child while feeling so terrible. She has been reasonably good, but it is difficult just to get up in the morning, let alone to play with a demanding toddler.

CANDY: What happened to you after the first few months, Rachel?

RACHEL: I have no other child to contend with, but I began having back trouble, and I couldn't even sit up for more than half an hour without raising my feet. It made me feel like an invalid. But the worst part of the pregnancy began at the end of my sixth month. I had difficulty breathing. It was really frightening. I felt as if I was suffocating. It turned out that I had asthma, but at the time I didn't know that. I kept going to my doctor, saying that I felt as if I needed oxygen, and he would just discount it. It was horrible to be gasping for breath and having the doctor tell me that there was nothing wrong, without even examining me.

BETH: I would like to add that I never had experienced sinus difficulties until I became pregnant. To this day I now have trouble with my sinuses. I think that there are a lot of physical changes that occur, and it's important to find out about them so that you don't think you're crazy.

CANDY: I had a great pregnancy, but I can see that I would have been completely unprepared for the psychological problems had they arisen. We all hear about morning sickness and eating crackers, but no one talks about women who feel disconnected from their children-to-be, or about becoming really upset and isolated from everyone. Given all the expectations, it must be incredibly disappointing.

RACHEL: Exactly. I had really assumed that those nine months were going to be the best of my life. Instead, they were the worst.

SARAH: During my first pregnancy I didn't get any support from my doctor. That made a bad pregnancy even more difficult. I finally went to and got help from a psychologist who specialized in pregnancy issues. She didn't really have any great suggestions, but she listened to and empathized with me. She validated that I was going through a stressful time.

RACHEL: The only person I could turn to for support was my husband. Although we had planned the pregnancy, once the initial euphoria wore off he became very anxious. He was afraid that both our relationship and his life were going to change, and he wasn't ready for that. He needed time to adjust, and he didn't have any because everything changed immediately. Since I was always sick, neither of us had a gradual transition to my being pregnant. I think that if I hadn't been sick it would have been easier, but as it was he couldn't deal with me at all. In fact he literally didn't talk to me for the first several months.

SARAH: During both my pregnancies I was so wrapped up in myself and my body that my husband's needs were totally secondary. I was self-absorbed and did not consider him at all. I remember thinking, the second time I became pregnant, that I was about to give up my body for eighteen months. That's really how I looked at it.

CANDY: If you have a good pregnancy, you don't think much about giving up your body. For me it was a healthy and happy time. I didn't think of it as a deprivation until the ninth month, when I did feel I wanted it to be over already. But for the first eight months, I felt together, attractive, and in control. I could concentrate on dealing with the baby who was coming.

RACHEL: That reminds me of a feeling I had. When I was at my sickest, I started praying that the baby would be premature. Even though I knew that would be risky, at those moments I cared only about me and getting better again.

BETH: That's the same as how I had wanted my labor to be natural, but when I was in such intense pain, I didn't care about the health of my baby. I cared only about me and stopping that pain. So I can understand what you are saying, even though I had an easy pregnancy.

CANDY: What was yours like, Beth?

BETH: I gained forty pounds. I wanted to start looking pregnant immediately, and my way of making that happen faster was to gain weight. Some of it was bound to reach my belly! I wanted to be this huge pregnant woman, and I was, but I wanted also to be extremely active. I wanted to have the best pregnancy in the world. I water-skied when I was in my sixth month, and cross-country skied when I was seven-months pregnant. People told me I was crazy, but I loved having them stare at me on the ski slopes. Because of this easy, healthy pregnancy, I imagined simply breezing through labor. I was dead wrong. From start to finish, it was a little over two days.

SARAH: Knowing what labor is really like makes this second pregnancy even more difficult. I have a hard time falling asleep, and I sometimes wake up thinking that labor was the worst pain I ever experienced in my life. I wonder what I am doing this again for.

CANDY: Why? Because our first children are so terrific, and there's such love that you can't help but want more. I feel that I should add that my labor was not bad at all, and not very painful. Believe it or not, you can have both a great pregnancy and great labor. Of course, I had a tough time with postpartum. I guess you can't have everything go your way.

BETH: I had three miscarriages between having my son and the pregnancy I'm now in. It was not easy. The first time I had a miscarriage it was very early; the second one happened later, at almost three months; and the third was very early again. I finally found out that I had a thyroid problem that was correctable. Although it was terrible having miscarriages, I think it was easier than having them *before* having had a child. I imagine that if I had miscarried before I had my son I would have feared I could never have a child. I went through a feeling of loss because I knew what it was that I had lost. But basically I was disappointed with my body — that it was not working right and naturally. I wasn't so afraid that I couldn't have another baby, which is the big fear with miscarriages.

RACHEL: I would like to add that in my ninth month, when most women can't wait for pregnancy to end, I started enjoying every day. I guess that was because I knew that there was an end in sight.

SARAH: The end of this pregnancy has been better than the end of my first one. When I heard that I might deliver early, a part of me said, Oh no, I may never be pregnant again. I'm not ready for it to end yet. But right now, two days *past* my due date, I've changed my mind.

MOTHERTALK is a group of new mothers who have been meeting monthly to discuss ways of dealing emotionally with certain issues raised by motherhood. Sometimes the meetings are animated and illuminating, but even when they are not, it is comforting and relaxing to sit around — without children or husbands — and feel the connectedness of being with other mothers.

Fears and Expectations

ROCHELLE BEAL

Nine-and-a-half months of pregnancy have not filled my mind with thoughts about babies. Actually, I'm pretty frightened of infants and politely decline all offers to hold them. What my pregnancy has done, however, is to affirm positive feelings about myself as a healthy, normal woman. Even now, two weeks past my "due date," I feel a wave of confidence when I realize that *I* was able to become pregnant.

Basically my pregnancy has been very pleasant. I have had no discomfort. My cheeks are a little rosier than usual, and my normally cold hands and feet have warmed up. I have always been five to ten pounds overweight, but never honest enough to admit those pounds were permanent. As a result, I would buy my clothes too tight in anticipation of losing the weight. With a new maternity wardrobe, this is the first time in a decade that my clothes actually fit properly. In fact, they are quite becoming. My formerly big hips look slender around the corner from my big belly. While I expected to regret this great loss of sexuality, I rather like being a cute, fat lady. By contrast, my husband is very concerned about my monthly weight gains and postpartum shape.

I've often heard women discussing the extra sensitivity and

13

moodiness they experience during pregnancy. For me it has been the exact opposite: I feel more grounded and less easily perturbed. Perhaps these feelings are connected with the immense relief I experienced at having passed a milestone around which I so strongly feared failure. Becoming pregnant, like getting married, was something I felt compelled to succeed at.

The immediacy of professional demands has prevented me from spending much time thinking about being pregnant. As comptroller of a mental health clinic, I am responsible for the entire financial functioning of the clinic. My job is totally absorbing; even when I am preparing an assignment at home, I become completely involved and ignore everything else. In fact, I have so much to accomplish before this baby arrives that I'm probably the only expectant mother who ever hoped that her child would be overdue. During the past few days, with the baby already one week late, I stayed cool as a cucumber. People think I'm amazingly patient. What they don't know is that every morning I wake up grateful that I have another day to polish off items on my "things-to-do" list.

———————

When I allow myself to think about the future, I worry about whether I'll love my child enough and whether I'll be a good mother. New-mother friends have told me that the moment they saw their infants, they were completely overwhelmed by the miracle of it all and felt instantaneous love. Being a quiet, undemonstrative type myself, I am quite certain that I will react neither that strongly nor that suddenly. But will deep feelings develop eventually? Will a gradually emerging love be adequate?

It seems incredible that my life is about to change dramatically, and yet I can't really envision how. Friends have been communicative about their birth experiences and have given me a good understanding of what to expect, but I have great difficulty imagining what is involved in actually caring for and loving a child. I hear about "maternal instinct" as though a good fairy flies down to every new mother and sprinkles special maternal dust on her. All I know is that I have not had much luck with house plants I have tended. I hope my performance level with a child is better than with my plants, and that babies are more resilient than coleus.

I have also lapsed into fears about having an unhealthy baby.

Although the statistics are in my favor, what if this is the time that I get paid back for those instances when I was mean or snide to someone? I cannot decide if I'm a lucky or unlucky person. Working in the immediate area of a children's hospital serves only to feed my worst fears. Every few days I see parents bringing their handicapped children into the hospital. The parents seem untormented by their lot in life. How can they possibly cope so well? I refused a baby shower at work because I would be too ashamed if my child were not normal. Also, it seemed like tempting fate to accept gifts before the birth.

During pregnancy you are supposed to sit back and relax. But throughout my life I've always worked extremely hard for the things I wanted, never relaxing. I simply cannot believe that my child will be normal if I'm not driving myself and preparing intensively in some manner.

When my husband and I attended childbirth classes, I hung on to every word the instructor said, excited that I would be using this information within a short time. Although I usually work hard for what I want, I *hate* exercising, and the breathing techniques have been a drag to practice. Mark is so eager that I sometimes feel we're preparing for the Olympics. We have developed a routine that begins with Mark suggesting early in the evening that we begin exercising. I cleverly delay with a variety of excuses. His obvious disappointment makes me feel like a bad mother even before my baby is born. Then I weigh my guilt against my dislike of exercising, and we end up practicing about every third night.

Despite my fears, I've thoroughly enjoyed the past nine months plus. I cherish my new sense of self as a normal, healthy woman. And perhaps after the baby is born I'll continue to buy clothes that actually fit me.

ROCHELLE BEAL is comptroller at a mental health clinic in Boston. After a four-month leave of absence, she has returned to work on a part-time basis.

2

Postpartum Changes

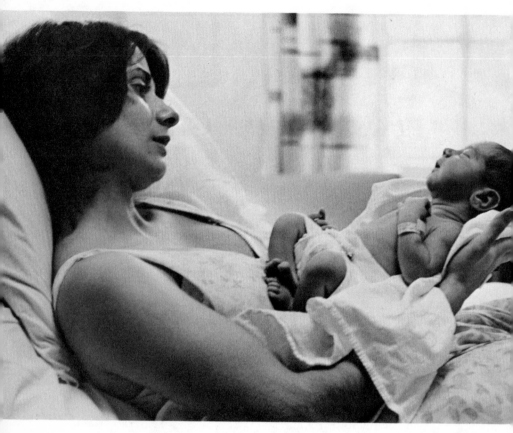

Ellen Shub

The First Six Months

MAUREEN X. O'BRIEN

Women are warned that becoming a mother means change. For me, this is cruel understatement. I lost my career, my independence, and my identity. Motherhood meant falling, crashing, building anew. It was like sculpting rock with fingernails.

From the beginning, I was beset by feelings of inadequacy. A helpless human being needed me for survival — limited, flawed, selfish me, who had always chafed at claims on my energy by anyone else. During my hospital stay, I felt overwhelmingly apologetic: to the staff for having "failed" at natural childbirth; to my roommates, who nicknamed my daughter "The Bitch" and who held out their placid babies like reproaches; and to Meg for those first stirrings of resentment when even my best efforts seemed fated to fail.

My first attempts at breast-feeding were chaotic. The nurse would hand me the baby, who was already wailing and clench-fisted, stare at my clumsy efforts to force a union between nipple and mouth, then descend on us like a hag, wrenching and tugging, pinching and prodding, until I was bathed in sweat and Meg's protests had awakened every baby on the floor.

At least being home meant privacy, familiar surroundings, and a chance to become better acquainted with my daughter. She began nursing well, and charmed me completely despite her erratic sleeping habits and a face swamped by nose and devoid of chin. But after the first few weeks of celebrity status as a new mother, sleepless nights began to take their toll, and I felt empty. Colorless day replaced colorless day: tedious, bleak, exhausting, uniform. All these words apply, but none conveys the terror.

For one thing, I became totally dependent on my husband, John, for my nurturing, a demand which I knew imperiled both our relationship and my self-respect. When he left in the morning, it was as if he took with him my ability to function.

I couldn't make the simplest decision. I would put Meg in for her morning nap, pour a cup of coffee, grab my smokes, and exult: an hour of freedom! Should I wash my hair? Yes. No. I might not have time to dry it. Should I wash those scummy dishes piled high on the kitchen counters? No. Rattling silverware never failed to wake the baby. Vacuum? Out of the question. Launder? Read? Write? Exercise? Call my mother? Pluck my eyebrows?

I practiced the same litany every day, my panic rising as the minutes passed, the options spinning faster and faster around in my head until, incredibly, I'd hear Meg gurgle, be shaken out of my stupor, and realize that I had spent the entire time staring out the window, poisoning my system with nicotine. The morning was shot, the house was a mess, and I was still in my stinking robe.

There were productive days and tender moments, but more typical were the days when I would run out of toilet paper, bread, and dogfood, and be incapable of finding solutions to these problems. If someone dropped in on such a day, I would wither in humiliation. I would see through their eyes the thick frosting of dog hair on the carpet and imagine them looking disapprovingly at my eyebrows, which threatened to engulf my nose. Serving coffee became a complex task. Trembling, I would search for two clean cups, hoping that the milk hadn't soured and wondering whether I could surreptitiously pick the coffee granules out of the sugar bowl. The kitchen table would be cluttered, and I would get an uncontrollable urge to knock the swill off with a sweep of my forearm. Conversation was impossible because I was too busy praying that my guest wouldn't have to go to the bathroom, and that I would be spared the mortification of having to supply paper napkins in lieu of the missing roll of toilet paper.

Worse still were the slow-motion days. I would think, This day is never going to end. No matter what I do or how slowly I do it, this day will last an eternity. I would become both an actress in a slow-motion film and a spectator. The game was to set an impossibly long time in which to complete a given task — five minutes, for example, to pick up a scrap of paper. I was trying to cheat time, but whenever I checked the clock, never did any activity take as much time as I had hoped. Then the spectator half of me would jeer like a disappointed fan, and I would go even slower still.

On one such day, as I was on the verge of losing control, I called a friend and begged her to come over. When she told me that she couldn't make it, I burst into tears. Somehow I survived the afternoon. John was due home any minute; I kept pacing and stealing glances out the window, willing his car to pull into the driveway. Then the phone rang. It was John calling to say that he was out drinking with friends. Though astounded by his defection, I said nothing. I simply decided that I would leave him and give him custody of the baby. I was very serious. Then I got very drunk.

I realized that chemical escapes were ultimately self-defeating, but the realization didn't stop me. Two drinks guaranteed insomnia and awful nights of bolting upright in bed, instantly alert, like a spy in danger. My mind would turn into a scanner that reviewed the day's events until a mistake was detected and flushed out of hiding. I would savor, suck on, and chew that mistake, then spit it out. But relief was short-lived and sleep impossible. The scanner would start up again and again until I silently implored Meghan to wake up and distract me from my self-flagellation.

In addition to the conclusion that I was an inept housewife and that I was becoming emotionally unraveled, I berated myself with the observation that I had lost my looks. I woke up groggy. My hair was mangled by mysterious night sweats, and my unwieldy breasts hung out of the gap in my old robe spotted white with spit-up. I can only imagine what John thought of greeting this apparition each morning, but the reflection in the mirror filled me with self-loathing.

I was fifteen pounds overweight, and gravity took on a new dimension. Of course I knew that dieting and exercise were the answer, but I did them only sporadically, on "up" days, after a hundred pep talks. I lost the same five pounds ten times during the first six months at home. Anyway, I rationalized, who ever saw me?

I refused to subject myself to the torture of buying new clothes and felt that I didn't deserve a haircut. But the ultimate in self-neglect came when I developed an infected cyst on my face, which dwarfed my other features. It was so grotesque that total strangers handed me the names of their dermatologists. Despite my husband's prompting, I merely watched with a kind of horrible fascination as it swelled and festered until so much scar tissue had accumulated that it could only be corrected by plastic surgery.

Although most of my anger was turned inward, some managed to seep out. I couldn't handle anger; it seemed so inappropriate. As a mother, I had expected to feel fulfilled, serene. More important, I could find no way to defuse my anger. Joking didn't work: there was no one around to laugh. Witty observations, saved for hours and hoarded for days, sounded shrill, out of context, laced with hysteria. Spilling my guts out failed too: there was no confessor available when I needed one. Ill-timed expressions of pain, groping and inarticulate, were interpreted as simple whining. A casual "How's the baby?" brought on tangled, self-pitying responses. People eventually stopped asking.

When I was the cheerful, sympathetic friend with patient ears and terrific eye contact, people couldn't leave me alone. During my crisis, they managed to do exactly that. It seemed that no one understood the nature of my pain; I certainly didn't understand their responses. My childless friends seemed smug and self-congratulatory, as if I were saying "Motherhood stinks," instead of "I'm in trouble."

My friends with children, on the other hand, were either amused or regarded me as a heretic. Obviously I was a mutant, a woman unhappy doing something for which she was biologically and culturally destined. An irritated mother friend once told me, "You're not the first person in the world to have a baby. Everyone else seems to manage." Exactly. That was the problem.

─────────

I was unhappy with the condition, but it by no means followed that I was unhappy with the baby. She evoked in me a concoction of intense emotions. Delight and despair shared the same space; jealousy with love; boredom with fascination; frustration with tranquillity. Meghan brought with her unexpected smiles, sweet smells, sudden laughter, and a chance to share innocence, discovery, and unlimited potential. She also brought unceasing demands, exhaustion, and imprisonment. She made me feel like the most significant person in the world, and the least important.

While Meg was good-natured, alert, and growing more beautiful each day, the exact reverse was true for me. She blossomed; I withered. Her world grew; mine diminished. She was rude: her cries shattered concentration, halted projects, and disrupted our gallant but doomed attempts to entertain. She was an ingrate: she saved all her smiles for her father and gave me red, contorted faces as she searched for my nipple or announced a soiled diaper. She was imperfect, sleeping poorly at night. She developed acne, and I had to endure suggestions that my milk was too rich or my sheets too dirty.

But Meg was also assertive, healthy, and bright. I was reluctant to keep this information to myself, and, like a stage mother, I showed her off as if she were a trained flea. What pleasure her performance brought me; her progress justified my very existence. I blissfully ignored cues that her audiences were alternately bored silly or resentful. I even looked forward to going to the pediatrician. My excitement would build the week before the appointment. I would select our outfits with painstaking care, scrub and iron, rehearse and primp. I was obviously hoping for a few crumbs of praise from some harried guy who had neither the time nor the desire to canonize me. Then I would lament anew at how narrow my world had become.

If I sometimes felt that Meghan flourished at my expense, John must have felt that my survival depended upon his daily energy transfusions. John is sexy, intelligent, courteous, and sensitive. Before becoming parents, we had spent seven years establishing a sweet and steady rhythm to our lives. People marveled at our compatability, our shared interests, and our deep commitment to each other. But when the baby was born, it was as if a siren had gone off during a performance of Beethoven. We became actors ad-libbing in a slapstick comedy: bumping into walls, slipping on banana peels, throwing pies in each other's faces. The frenzy to adjust exerted considerable strain on our relationship. But we tried. Boy, did we try.

John went to work exhausted. Although I got up with the baby three times a night, he wasn't deaf: Meg cried as if an ax murderer were in the crib with her. He'd come home to a sloppy house and a sloppier wife, who would be poised at the door waiting to dump some emotional baggage on him. After counseling on his job for eight hours, he would be forced to counsel me. Ever patient, he listened and consoled.

Then he took over total care of the baby. He fed, bathed, and soothed her, and he treated her diaper rash. His shoulders got just as wet with drool as mine did. It is no accident that Meg now prefers him. He has earned her love.

————

Now that I am back working, I understand the scope of his sacrifice. At the time I was grateful but felt entitled. Therein lies a conflict: his sacrifice was immense; I was entitled. Both statements are true. We were drowning in chores and working so hard; yet no matter how hard we tried, it never seemed enough. Someone always felt cheated.

Rules gradually changed. General complaints, such as "This is the pits," or "Only seventeen-and-a-half more years to go," were allowed. But specific complaints — "You should know by now where her rubber pants are kept," or "Just one day I'd like to come home and be able to find a clean spoon" — created swift and devastating results. Through the duration of our marriage John and I had been very civilized combatants. Now we were fighting continuously, and there were no limitations imposed.

Insults became part of the arsenal. John's were as painful as knife wounds, mostly because they forced me to look at the person I had become. Once I had been feisty under attack. Now I couldn't retreat fast enough — behind the couch, curled in the fetal position, or lying in bed, arms folded across my chest, whimpering, thirsting for a touch.

Although John denies it, he began to avoid coming home. It suddenly became essential for him to wait around for three hours after work to play in a basketball game that lasted forty-five minutes; or to stop off for a drink with his colleagues, which lasted through supper. He was my lifeline and I reacted to these retreats like an ogre. He was looking for room to breathe, and I was holding onto him by the ankles.

Our sex life changed. We made love less frequently, but there was an urgency, a physicality, a new dimension to sex that erased the boredom and irritation and reaffirmed our love.

Despite the upheaval and the pain, John and I never lost confidence in the ability of our relationship to withstand any assault. Despite our self-protective posturing and me-first impulses, we always kept an eye open for the other's well-being. John rescued me a hundred times by making me feel beautiful when I was ugly;

planting an unexpected kiss on my forehead; cracking a well-timed joke. He more often than not was able to reach out and give when, by rights, he shouldn't have had anything left.

Things started falling into place around the six-month mark. Spring arrived. Meg started sleeping through the night. I stopped nursing. I went on a diet. Meg became a person. I was suddenly ready to make some decisions. I decided that I was no housewife and that I would return to teaching. It was not easy to part with my myth: I very much wanted to be one of those attractive suburban mothers, delighted to devote all her time to handsome children and household projects. But I recognized that I had different needs and that trying to meet these needs could only have a beneficial effect on my family. In other words, I decided that what made me happy would make everybody else happy, an admittedly selfish conclusion. My final realization is that selfishness is terribly underrated.

MAUREEN X. O'BRIEN returned to teaching when her daughter was a year old. Meg stays with a neighbor and friend in Scituate, Massachusetts, where the O'Briens live.

A New Mother's Journal

SIMONE BLOOM

The Hospital

My baby girl was born yesterday. The pain is still with me, but I am floating on a delicious high with the realization that she is alive, healthy, and the beginning of a whole new life.

Despite expectations, I felt no instant bonding when she was born. It bothered me to admit it, but I really didn't want to be with her at that moment. I felt sheer relief that my ordeal, and the physical and emotional exhaustion, were over at last. I held her briefly and heard her cry, but my surroundings of bright lights, doctors, and medical equipment, combined with being on my back with feet up in stirrups, were not conducive to fostering initial maternal feelings. I just wanted to be totally by myself. However, as soon as I was being wheeled to my room, I immediately wanted to see my baby and put her to my breast. (I had been ambivalent about nursing, but after seeing my baby and holding her, there was no question in my mind. It was just the natural thing to do.)

I am in conflict: I am happy and I am sad; I need to talk and I need to be quiet; I need company and I need privacy; I want to share my infant and I want her all to myself. I am one day into motherhood.

———————

I cannot stop marveling at her perfect formation, her peaceful sleeping face, and her shock of black hair. I feel awkward and uncomfortable about handling her, but I am learning. I hate to hear her cry. I want to cradle and comfort her whenever she does.

I am slowly getting over the childbirth experience. I am talking it through and working it through, and in spite of my "episiotomy shuffle," I am recovering. I enjoy talking with the first-time mothers, comparing labors and babies. When I talk with another mother, I immediately dismiss those who have other children. This experience is too unique to share with those who have already been through it.

———————

I have made a friend. Her baby was born on the same day as mine. We take names and addresses and promise to keep in touch. Being in the hospital does not allow me much free time. I go to a breast-feeding class; as I return, the phone rings. Jennifer is wheeled in crying to be fed; the phone keeps ringing; my lunch arrives. When the doctor pops in, I am embarrassed at my exposed breast. The baby will not suckle. I feel an increasing frustration because my milk has not come in. Why won't she suckle? She must be punishing me because I had negative feelings toward her today. I feel very overwhelmed by the jumble of emotions I am experiencing.

Time to Go Home

The nurse brings Jennie to my husband and me, and we gingerly dress her. It is raining outside. We proudly walk to the car and get in. I am anxious, but delighted about returning home. Everything has been prepared and Jennie goes straight to sleep. I slowly get into bed and luxuriate in the silence around me.

The visitors start arriving — just immediate family. They take pictures and watch Jennie nurse. My husband puts his arm protectively around me and shares in the nursing experience. We watch her expression of contentment as she suckles. We burp her, bathe her, and change her diapers.

———

The night feedings are exhausting. Two or three times during the night I am up. I often feel a spiritual communion with all the other mothers who are feeding their babies in the still of the night. Jennie is a good baby. She mostly eats and sleeps, and I nurse her whenever she cries. But she is starting to get fussy at night. She screams; then I cannot comfort her. I try everything. I jiggle her, rock her, sing to her, and lie on the couch with her. She will not stop crying. I get angry. I wonder why I ever decided to have a baby. I regret the decision. I want her to stop screaming, and my tolerance wears thin. Eventually I disintegrate into tears, and my husband finds us both on the floor, weeping and wailing. He comforts us both and puts us back to bed, saying tomorrow will be better.

I am learning to take naps. I can fall asleep very quickly and do so at every available opportunity. My friend from the hospital calls me. We talk incessantly about every minute detail of our babies' activities. It is good to talk to someone in the same boat. The U.P.S. truck brings presents. It is exciting to open them all, and I am starting to make a collage of all the cards. I appreciate every single one of them; having a baby makes me feel a general closeness with humanity.

———

Where does time go? I feel helpless as days pass me by and I cannot manage to do more than care for my baby. I am grateful for frozen quiches, Kentucky Fried Chicken, and any contribution of snacks;

I miss all the time I used to have to cook. No full-time job was ever as demanding as this, and the rewards are minimal. I am slowly getting into some sort of routine as I learn that the byword of these first weeks is *while* — do it while you can, be it taking a shower, making a phone call, washing clothes, or whatever. I have abandoned any attempts at housecleaning and have reconciled myself to dust balls under the couch and piles of unanswered correspondence.

Every mother I know has suddenly been elevated to heroine in my mind. I had no idea what they all went through to raise their families! I feel a special closeness toward my own mother, even though she is literally at the other end of the world.

————

My relationship with my husband is tense. We are both reveling in our baby, but she is putting severe strains upon us. We are constantly interrupted with cries, feedings, or diarrhea, and we don't even seem to have a chance for a quiet dinner together. I am becoming quite skilled at one-handed eating as I find myself nursing Jennie through dinner. Why does she have to get cranky at dinnertime? There seems to be no time for conversation, and as for sex, it is the farthest thing from our minds right now. Will our relationship ever be the same again? I worry, but something tells me things will work out. One thing, however, is clear to me. No matter how much we thought we were prepared for this, with a solid and tested marriage behind us, childbirth education, financial security, and endless reading, the reality of having a newborn is inconceivable beforehand.

Two Weeks
It is late September. I decide it is time for Jennifer and me to venture out into the world. I rig up my front sling, and we set out for the supermarket. I enjoy the feeling of having my baby so close to my body — of her heartbeat and her little doe eyes peering up at me. I feel a rush of loving warmth as we walk. I am amazed (and secretly delighted) at how many people stop me to have a look at my baby. Motherhood seems to break all social barriers as conversations with strangers of all ages and backgrounds evolve. I feel a special kinship

with anyone who has an infant, stopping to discuss age, weight, sleeping habits, and diapers. Six-month-old babies look huge to me, and I cannot imagine that Jennie will ever be that big. In much the same way that I noticed every pregnant woman I saw when I was pregnant, I am drawn to *every* baby I see. I feel a great need to share my experience, and I find myself contacting acquaintances who have babies, just to talk. I feel very much apart from my friends who do not have children. When talking with a former workmate, I realize that my entire conversation has been about my daughter. I remember how I used to find it irritating and boring when people did that to me. But, at the moment, my whole existence revolves around my daughter and her needs, and it really is the only thing that interests me.

A concerned friend suggests that my husband and I go out to dinner alone. We are unable to leave our baby, especially not with some strange baby sitter. We want to nurture her; she is so tiny and dependent. My husband, who never liked children much, confessed that when he rocked Jennifer to her first night's sleep and felt her clinging desperately "like a little monkey" to him, all his reservations melted away. Now he is truly besotted with his daughter. He is very involved in her care, and can't wait to get home at night to see her. I snapped a picture of the two of them — Jennie peacefully sleeping on his chest as he slept. It is so nice to see this side of him reveal itself.

Three Weeks

Jennie smiled for the first time — a gentle parting of her lips into a contented, happy crinkle, and we are filled with delight and excitement. We get out her baby book and make the first notation.

Things have settled down somewhat. My sense of bewilderment is fading as I begin to assimilate the incredible changes we have gone through. The most difficult thing to cope with is constant exhaustion, and I am eagerly awaiting the magical night when Jennie sleeps through.

I feel like patting myself on the back merely for surviving the past weeks. There is no question that they have been the most overwhelming, exciting, difficult, and disruptive of my life. *Nothing* compares to or prepares one for the changes. These first three weeks have been very special. They are the beginning of a new life as a family, not a couple, and of learning to put someone else's needs before our own.

    SIMONE BLOOM was twenty-five when her daughter was born. Simone was born and educated in Johannesburg, South Africa, and lived and worked in Australia before settling in the Boston area. She plans to work once her two children are in school.

Surviving Colic . . . Twice

TERESA VERCOLLONE CRYAN

I can picture myself, plump and sleepy-eyed, sitting up expectantly and listening for the cries of my first-born as he was wheeled down the corridor from the nursery. Although I had to search for the name sign on his crib to recognize my own by sight, within three days I could distinguish his cry from the tangle of others. And it seemed that he was always crying.

    Perhaps I should have known then. But, in fact, it wasn't until the three difficult months had long passed that I allowed myself to put a label on the misery that had ruled our lives — colic. With my second colicky baby, however, I recognized the symptoms — and named them — immediately. Most experts, while disagreeing on the causes of colic, point to tension in the environment as a major contributing factor. Thus, no matter where you turn, the result is guilt: you are causing your defenseless infant and yourself three months of unnecessary misery.

    By refusing to label the fussiness of my first child, I was simply blocking out that guilt. I realize now that this blocking approach was possible only because his case of colic was mercifully mild.

    From the beginning, Stephen's distress was erratic. There

would be good mornings followed by miserable afternoons, agonizing days interspersed with quiet evenings, peaceful hours on the heels of horrible sieges. His colic never developed a pattern, such as the fussy late afternoons and evenings many colicky babies suffer.

For the first two weeks at home, I shared baby care with my husband and then my mother. Because two adults could spell each other during the sporadic fussy periods, they passed by almost unnoticed. In fact, at Stephen's second-week checkup, the nurse asked me if he was troubled by gas. I responded honestly, "Not that I've noticed."

The next week, alone at home with baby, I noticed. We weathered a few intermittent "bad" periods early in the week. On Thursday morning, I nursed and burped him, careful to squeeze out every last bubble, and gently laid him down. He fell into a peaceful sleep, only to awaken twenty minutes later in fitful agony. There were three or four replays of this scene, and, by the end of the afternoon, his cries had built to frantic, frightening squalls. He would screw his hands into fists, clutch his legs tight to his body, wring his face into a distorted mask, and wail.

The maneuvers that usually soothed the savage beast didn't put a dent in the cries this time. Finally, I hit upon the cure: jogging around the living room in time to music. But the cure took as much out of me as the malady, and by five o'clock we were sitting at the kitchen table in tears — Stephen in his infant seat and I slumped in a chair, alternately pleading and swearing.

This was the scene that greeted my husband when he poked his head through the door, and, quite literally, caught the baby that I tossed to him. We passed Stephen back and forth for the next two hours until he finally fell into a deep sleep, slung over Peter's knee.

Miraculously, most of Stephen's fussiness could be soothed with a pacifier. I had always found the sight of babies chomping on that artificial, plastic nipple decidedly distasteful. But I didn't realize that few newborns could comfort themselves by reliably bringing their hands to their mouth, never mind inserting a finger. Once we discovered the amazing abilities of pacifiers, there were several pacifiers in every room of the house, three in my pocketbook, and a few in the glove compartment of the car. And it was, in fact, that little bit of plastic that got our baby through those bad periods and often saved our sanity.

31

When the "attacks" (as we began to call them) interrupted Stephen's sleep, we would prop him up in the infant seat and stick in the pacifier. He would suck furiously during an attack — the tempo of his sucking seemed to match the intensity of the pain — then drop off into a limp sleep for ten minutes. This alternating pattern of pain and brief naps could continue for hours.

Stephen's fussiness seemed to peak at six weeks and then recede rapidly. By the second month, we could nap together and both get some sleep, albeit interrupted. By three months, the attacks were infrequent and involved relatively little wailing. By six months, he had blossomed into an easygoing baby with a remarkably sunny disposition — the kind of baby you could plop down on the kitchen floor to amuse himself for twenty minutes; the kind of baby who could be passed around at family gatherings and retain his friendly equanimity. Rather than being the sensitive, active, high-strung child described in the literature on colicky infants, he seemed to be the exact opposite.

It was only then — when I had living proof that there was nothing wrong with my mothering — that I began to speculate about the possibility of colic.

I discovered that there are many theories about colic, but few certainties. The array of findings and opinions about its causes convinced me that the jury is still out. So when our second baby, Phillip, came down with the symptoms, I was able to diagnose and accept the malady with regret, but without guilt.

For the first two weeks, Phillip was a model infant, nursing enthusiastically, burping promptly, and sleeping peacefully. Just as I was daring to believe that I had been rewarded with an "easy" baby, colic struck.

It was his two-week birthday, and my sister was escorting Stephen on a heady afternoon of McDonald's and the Children's Museum. I planned to spend the entire day in my bathrobe after popping Phillip into bed for his dependable two-hour nap.

After the midmorning feeding, I confidently settled him into his bassinet. Screams. I covered all the usual checkpoints, from pins to rashes, and put him back to bed. But those screams had a certain desperate and strangely familiar quality to them. I nursed him again . . . and again . . . and again. He never did get back into the bassinet and, at three that afternoon, I was tripping with fatigue around the house in time to James Taylor.

This colic, as it turned out, was the real thing. While his attacks, like Stephen's, came sporadically, the good times were briefer. And he was consistently more miserable in the evening. His distress (and ours) was intensified by his adamant refusal of the pacifier, thus negating one major way of getting himself (and us) through the pain.

But while the colic was more severe, the mother was more experienced, less guilty, and more willing to identify the problem and search for practical solutions, from reclining naps and extensive use of a swing to cutting out milk products in my diet.

Although all these techniques were helpful, they didn't provide a cure. Colic still ruled our days and ruined many of them. And colic still placed a tremendous strain on our marriage.

Having a baby, especially the first, brings stress to any marital relationship. Having a colicky baby, especially the first, intensifies that stress. Even without the imposing views of experts, the primary caretaker's self-image is bound to take a beating, simply because a colicky baby seems terribly unhappy. That insecurity, plus the sheer fatigue from waltzing around with six pounds on your shoulder, can gnaw away at the most serene marriage.

Peter and I were both terminally exhausted, on edge, and frustrated. Peter was less than anxious to come home each evening (though he always did), and I was more jealous of the relative calm he enjoyed at the office. Somehow we not only weathered the storm (twice), but came through with a galvanized sense of togetherness — somewhat akin to the exhilaration of people who battle a crisis together and win.

Even though Peter was away most of the day, when he stepped in the door, we shared — literally handing the baby back and forth all evening. Usually we both stayed up until the last bell was sounded — until we could deposit that sleeping bundle in the crib, tiptoe out, and fall into our own bed.

I've noticed other new parents, with easy babies, sparring over who will hold the infant during its brief periods out of the crib. Typically the father hangs in the background, waiting for his wife to finish nursing so that he can cuddle the baby. Our colicky babies were *always* awake and *always* needed holding, and I was always delighted to pass them off to another pair of arms.

The parents of colicky babies need solidarity in the face of still another stress: the well-meaning advice that comes from all sides. Everybody has a theory about what's wrong with your baby and what you should do about colic. We were the recipients of lots of useless hints on how to burp, how to hold, and how to tell if you have enough milk (because surely this baby isn't getting enough, even though it's gaining beautifully). The only people whose personal experience makes them qualified to advise you are the parents of colicky babies. Interestingly, they are the only people who don't.

We never found another weary couple whose baby's bout with colic coincided with ours, but older friends who had survived colic twenty years ago understood. They didn't get nervous when we ate dinner to the accompaniment of baby wails; neither did they become disoriented when we tried to carry on a conversation while jogging around the kitchen, nor did they grab for the baby, certain that their expert handling would soothe the cries. When the infant was handed to them, they unconsciously used little holding and rocking techniques that calmed him. They didn't offer any advice; they just sighed a lot and smiled sympathetically.

Their sympathy was not for the baby, but for us: while the baby is sure to come through colic with equanimity, the parents are at more risk. Common-sense techniques help, but they don't cure the colic or the mother's distress. In the final analysis, the most powerful sanity saver for us was the knowledge that colic comes to an end. I circled Phillip's three-month birthday on the calendar in bright red and crossed off each day we survived. By the time we hit that magic circle, what had emerged was an adorable, affectionate (from all that holding?) baby — a baby I felt was our just reward for three months of colic.

TERESA VERCOLLONE CRYAN, freelance writer and public relations consultant, became a mother at thirty. "I was astounded that a thirty-year-old woman can be brought weeping to her knees by a three-week-old bundle of joy. But I was equally amazed that a person I'd known only a few brief weeks could touch me so profoundly."

Triplets

AVRIL F. NAJMAN

The news that I was going to give birth to triplets left my husband and me absolutely thrilled. Without a second thought for any of the difficulties — physical, emotional, and financial — which we have since encountered, we sailed headlong into disaster with grins on our faces and a set of highly unrealistic, romantic notions about parenting.

The first change came four weeks before the children were born, when I was hospitalized as a safety precaution because I was carrying a triple load. Going into the hospital six weeks before the expected birth date instantly killed some of the romanticism. Simply being in the hospital was disruptive: it put me in a sick role. I was treated as a patient and very soon adapted to that role. Also, many women in the antenatal ward were indeed medically in jeopardy and were very anxious about the future well-being of their babies. Their anxiety was contagious, and I became depressed.

Bored and miserable, I closed my mind to the possibility that I might require a Caesarean section because of the way the babies were lying. I counted so much on a natural delivery that I could not cope with the surgery when it did indeed become necessary. When I came round from the anesthetic, I had no interest in my children and only felt sore and sorry for myself. When I finally saw them a full day later there was no sudden feeling of inner joy and love. They were just three more babies behind a glass screen in the premature nursery. I did feel distressed at seeing the smallest of the three being tube-fed, but seeing any baby being tube-fed would have upset me.

Getting over the operation, where all the others around me had babies to care for while I lay back with nothing to do except feel sorry for myself, was further depressing. I continually felt unhappy. I had little contact with my children during that time. While my physical needs and those of my children were carefully attended to, emotional needs were totally neglected.

The final blow came when I was discharged from the hospital, nearly three weeks after giving birth, with only one child. I felt cheated. Trying to fit in hospital visits (I felt obliged to go although I was not allowed to hold babies), along with caring for a new baby at home, was exhausting. The overtiredness only served to make a bad situation worse. The second daughter came home before she was four weeks old, and our son was home by five weeks. It was the beginning of our life as a family; however, it was also the beginning of the most stressful period of our lives.

⸻⸻⸻

The ill-conceived notions about parenting that I had entertained made motherhood even more difficult than it needed to be. I had imagined that no job was too burdensome to undertake for one's children, that patience should be unending, and that exhaustion could not possibly prevent me from attending lovingly to all their needs. And of course I expected them always to be happy, contented babies. I felt that for triplets I should give up my personal existence and commit myself to their care as a labor of love.

I attributed my infants' less-than-perfect behavior to failings in my own character and mothering. I had given up my outside life and life inside the home became exhausting, monotonous, and boring. The weight of responsibility was overwhelming. As far as I am concerned, it was pure hard work and frustration. I remember one occasion when I felt so miserable and unhappy that I began to weep. But I couldn't afford even the luxury of lying on my bed and crying it out of my system: I had to keep washing and preparing bottles. I remember feeling like a martyr, and I neglected almost everything except the children's physical needs. I rarely resented the children; I believed that the rut I was in must be normal, and so I began to accept it.

⸻⸻⸻

One of the most frustrating aspects of my children's infancy was not being able to give myself wholly to any one of them. Attending to one inevitably meant that the other two would try to attract my attention by behaving in some manner that would inevitably distress me. This made me angry, and I would subsequently not attend to any of them. Then, of course, I would feel guilty. The major individualized attention that each child received was in the care of their physical needs, such as changing nappies* and bathing. Even feeding was not very personal, because the triplets were frequently propped with a bottle while I winded† each one in succession.

My relationship with my husband also changed during the early years of being a mother. There were times when I had unrealistic expectations of him and times when I felt he had unrealistic expectations of me. Inevitably the days when he had had a particularly bad time at work and came home exhausted were the same days when I could least cope and felt that he should be attending to me and to the children. Sometimes I blamed myself for being inadequate, both as a mother and a wife, and other times I blamed my husband for not carrying his share of the load. Looking back, I realize that we were both stretched beyond our capacity to cope.

Things began to change when the children were about three years old. By then they could verbalize some of their needs and were sufficiently independent to reduce their demands on me. But I still felt guilty at not having the time to give each child individual love and affection. I regret that my children have had to compete for parental affection, that they had to share their love from the beginning. They have never had a unique place in the family as single infants do. On the the other hand, they have a "specialness" which lies in their being triplets; it has had its good and bad points for them.

If I have painted a dismal picture, it is because that is how it really was: infancy was a nightmare. There were times when I simply did not want the responsibility of caring for three. There were times when I went to bed thinking that I had not said a kind word to them all day. Things which may be cute and only occasionally frustrating in one are unbearable and exhausting in three. I have no desire to have another baby.

But as the children have grown older, the change for the better has snowballed, and the joys and pleasures of triplets now seem to be not three but one hundred times better than the pleasures of

* Diapers (in Australia, where the Najmans live)
† Burped

having only one could ever be. This does not mean that it has been straight sailing since they turned from infants to toddlers. But as the demands have altered, I have found them easier to cope with. I have also come to realize that most of our reactions were perfectly normal, and that our babies behaved much the same as any others. I still find the inevitable vying for attention somewhat frustrating, especially when they are trying to tell me about something that happened while they were away from me, and it is immediately spoiled for the two who cannot blurt it out first. But I see that this is normal behavior among any siblings rather than peculiar to triplets. I no longer believe it is a failing on my part.

After seven years, I am at last adjusting to motherhood and tripleting.

AVRIL F. NAJMAN had to contend with the shock of becoming an instant family of five, six hundred miles away from her family and friends. The Najmans live in Queensland, Australia.

3

Breast or Bottle

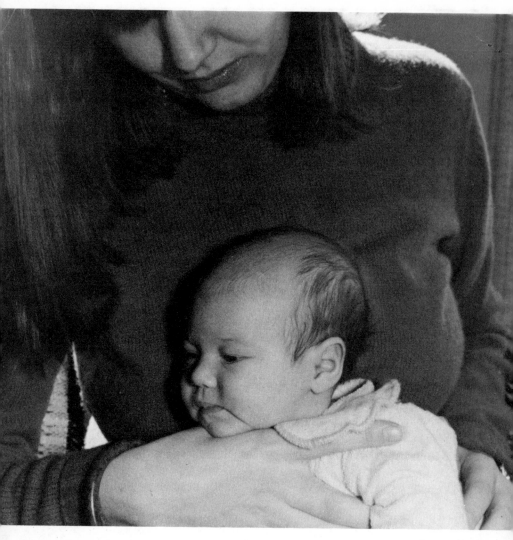

Joan Albert

Night Feeding

MURIEL RUKEYSER

Deeper than sleep but not so deep as death
I lay there sleeping and my magic head
remembered and forgot. On first cry I
remembered and forgot and did believe.
I knew love and I knew evil:
woke to the burning song and the tree burning blind,
despair of our days and the calm milk-giver who
knows sleep, knows growth, the sex of fire and grass,
and the black snake with gold bones.

Black sleeps, gold burns; on second cry I woke
fully and gave to feed and fed on feeding.
Gold seed, green pain, my wizards in the earth
walked through the house, black in the morning dark.
Shadows grew in my veins, my bright belief,
my head of dreams deeper than night and sleep.
Voices of all black animals crying to drink,
cries of all birth arise, simple as we,
found in the leaves, in clouds and dark, in dream,
deep as this hour, ready again to sleep.

Breast-Feeding

ANN D. BUNTING

If I had been asked to draw a self-portrait at certain moments during my nine months of breast-feeding, I would have drawn two large breasts and a vagina. These were the times, mostly early in the morning or late at night, when I felt torn apart: my child, my husband, and my own needs to have my body, time, and mind to myself exhausted me. Often weary, I felt guilty about the huge amount of physical attention I gave to my son, and equally guilty about my lack of physical interest in my husband. Only vaguely could I remember not being "on call" for an every-two-hours-hungry infant.

Fortunately, Bruce was very supportive and understanding of my breast-feeding. Being as tired and unsure as I was with new motherhood, nursing would not have been so satisfying had it not been for his caring attitude. He was comfortable with my feeding Logan anywhere, and in front of whoever was present.

Most people seemed to enjoy being with us while I nursed my son. But some, even close friends, were not entirely supportive. They questioned the nutritional value or my casualness or the length of time I continued to nurse. A few became uncomfortable and embarrassed over my nursing, refusing to look anywhere near me while we carried on a conversation.

———

My sister's child was born five days before Logan. Susan also nursed. She and Hadley flew from their home in Illinois to ours in North Carolina six weeks after the births of our children. The two of us sat on the front porch for long afternoons, nursing and rocking our children. During those moments of shared bonding with our infants, we also reaffirmed our bond as sisters.

One early morning, during this all-too-brief week together, I awoke to the sound of my child crying; then suddenly there was total quiet. Quickly I pulled myself out of bed and stumbled into the living room, which was on the way to Logan's bedroom. There, sitting on the couch, Susan was holding both children — Hadley suckling from one breast, Logan from the other.

———————

For the most part, I loved the experience nursing gave to me. I treasured the closeness, the importance, the cloud of warmth that enveloped my child and me when he suckled. On good days, it was one of the only times that I could picture myself as beautiful: the kind of beauty that comes from total giving, receiving, tenderness, and the certainty of being where I was most needed and loved. Together, my son and I were perfect; we were beautiful.

After nine months, my son refused to nurse. My breasts swelled painfully; my husband finally had to relieve the pressure since hand and breast pumps were too painful to use. Four days passed and still my child refused the breast. The last time he nursed was on the fourth "dry" night, when I caught him off guard. I took him from his crib, barely awake, and placed him to my breast. It worked; he suckled sleepily. Realizing that our nursing was indeed over, both relieved and saddened, I rocked and nursed him in the darkness long after I physically needed to.

I felt rejected and hurt when my child ended our nursing relationship. For several days, when he asked for a bottle I would simply hand it to him. Once I realized what I was doing, I felt both foolish and mean. I began holding and rocking him as he drank from his bottle. We regained our closeness. I let go a little of my hold, and our relationship grew in another direction. One period in our lives as mother and child had been completed.

ANN D. BUNTING lives in Wrightsville Beach, North Carolina, with her husband of five years and their son Logan. Her husband's two children from a previous marriage live with them part time. Ann worked at a mental health center before her son was born.

Working and Nursing

VICKY McMILLAN

The fact that I persisted in breast-feeding my daughter while continuing to work seemed to astonish many other women. I received considerable praise and admiration — compliments that I felt I hardly deserved since nursing seemed, to me, the only possible way I could juggle the demands of motherhood and a career. Looking back on my decision to breast-feed, I can see that I was driven by the need for perfection — to be both Supermother and Superbiologist — at least within the limits of my own definitions. The knowledge that I could leave the baby sitter bottles of breast milk — and thus part of myself — helped to lessen the tension between two conflicting parts of my life.

During my pregnancy, nursing had been the subject of many months of careful reading, discussions with other women, and solitary deliberation. Intellectually I was attracted to the idea: its nutritional and physical benefits seemed obvious. But although I was a biologist, the idea of nursing a baby myself seemed strange. I was more comfortable with the notion of bottle and formula. We live across from a dairy farm, and even the sight of milk-laden cows unsettled me: was I really destined for a role like that? I also did not believe the claims that nursing doesn't have to tie a mother down. The first few weeks, especially, sounded horrendous: how could I possibly feed a baby as often as every two hours, and do anything else?

Despite my eagerness to become a parent, and the joy with which I anticipated interacting with my child, I had no intention of neglecting other aspects of my life. Continuing in biology was vital to my sense of personal worth, even to my sanity. Friends had told me that it might take weeks to get a good nursing regime established, and I wasn't sure I wanted to make that sacrifice.

The decision to nurse was not an easy one, but in the end it was made spontaneously as I lay on the delivery room table and was given Jennifer, only a few minutes old, to hold in my arms. At that moment, nursing her seemed the most natural and logical thing to do. I remember thinking that it seemed to be so easy: all I had to do was lie there.

Although I was prepared for some pain from nursing, especially at first, I was lucky enough to experience almost no discomfort. My milk supply was more than adequate, and Jennifer was a capable, hearty eater. In fact, the act of nursing remained as effortless as it had been the first time in the delivery room. The greatest hardship was lack of sleep: I remember those first weeks as a blur of nights merging into days, my time and energy fractured by a seemingly endless stream of feedings. Sleep became the most precious commodity in the world. Rob helped with all aspects of Jennifer's care, and even got up with me for most night feedings; but I still felt exhausted. I had not realized how energy-depleting breast-feeding is, particularly at a time when the body is recovering from the rigors of childbirth. Valued parts of myself — spontaneity, creativity, musical and literary interests, a delight in good food and wine, and a sense of humor — were put aside during the first few months of Jennifer's life. I was bone-tired and harried, but efficient.

Although I had worked steadily throughout my pregnancy, even up to nine hours before Jennifer's birth, there were still several studies I needed to complete before the fall semester of teaching. I managed this with the help of Rob, who gave Jennifer bottles when I was absent for feedings. She accepted these readily. I established a routine of expressing milk and storing it in the sterilized, plastic bags that serve as bottles for Playtex nursers. It usually took about fifteen minutes to express enough milk for one feeding, and although I had no trouble in doing so, I found it a tedious chore and had to discipline myself to do it regularly.

One difficulty we experienced at this time was figuring out how much expressed milk to give at any one feeding. I will never forget the afternoon when I returned from one of my field sites and found Jennifer lying on Rob's lap looking absolutely bloated, as if she had been inflated like a balloon. Apparently she had been fretful after she finished her bottle, so Rob had thawed out another bag of milk and fed her some more. She still seemed hungry, so he had made another trip to the freezer for a third bottle. Within about half an hour, she drank nine-and-one-half ounces, a huge meal for a three-week-old baby.

This experience was one of many that demonstrated our initial inability to distinguish hunger cries from other sounds of distress. Even after we learned how, we worried about how much to put in a bottle. If we didn't put in enough, Jennifer would be crying with hunger while Rob frantically thawed out more milk, a process that seemed to take forever at such times. If we gave her too generous a serving, we had to throw out some of it; and I became increasingly sensitive to the sight of my precious hand-expressed milk disappearing down the drain.

Once our teaching duties resumed in September, we left Jennifer in the care of a baby sitter, along with bottles of breast milk and an emergency supply of formula. Since I was fortunate enough to have no classes on Tuesdays and Thursdays, I spent those days at home with Jennifer, doing what paperwork I could manage (usually not much). The rest of the work week, while I taught lectures and labs, I missed her very keenly. I continued to express milk on days that I was away from her, storing it in my usual little bags, and cooling them in an ice chest in my office until I left for home. The only difficulty here was finding the time: my days at work were always harried, and I sometimes missed a "feeding." This put me behind in my milk supplies and caused me physical discomfort. However, I remained committed to leaving breast milk with the baby sitter: it was an important symbol to me, and proof that I was not really abandoning my child. Although I realized the fallacies of such reasoning, continuing to provide breast milk without interruption was the crutch that I needed to cope with separations so early in the mother/child relationship.

Jennifer is now seven months, and I am still nursing, although we are also introducing solids. I avoid thinking about stopping nursing altogether: it has become a way of life, a means of creating a special closeness, and a convenience. I feel tremendous satisfaction in the knowledge that I can nourish my child myself without neglecting other obligations. I realize that fortunate circumstances have permitted this: a flexible schedule, work that allows me to be basically my own boss, no serious physical discomforts from nursing, and a husband who shares the chores and provides moral support even when he is as tired as I am. The most trying problem —

fatigue — is certainly aggravated by nursing, but it is difficult to say how much more tiring it would be to worry about bottles all the time. I am sure that I benefit from a reservoir of strength that comes from my pleasure in being able to feed my child in the manner that I wish.

VICKY McMILLAN is a biologist, the wife of a biologist, and the mother of a seven-month-old daughter. She and her family live in Poolville, New York.

Why I Prefer the Bottle

JOAN S. KLETZKER

My breast-feeding experience lasted exactly thirty-two days. I did not stop because my milk was slow to come in, because I was returning to work, or because I became ill. I put my baby on formula because I never really liked nursing. In fact, by the time I stopped I almost hated it. How could this be? Everyone had claimed that nursing would be a marvelous experience. But from day one, I found it terribly frustrating. I felt guilty, confused, disappointed, and resentful.

In all the current literature on new mothers, practically no support is given to the woman who opts not to nurse her child. I am not denying the importance of breast-feeding: I realize that it helps the mother's uterus contract to its normal size faster; and I realize that mother's milk is perfect for the baby because of the natural immunities. I certainly would never tell anyone not to nurse, but I think more attention should be paid to the mothers who have problems with it.

My first difficulty was with my nipples. In the hospital, I discovered that mine were inverted. As much as I tried, they never really came out. I attempted to get my baby to go to the breast several times, but to no avail. She was hungry and impatient and would not let nature do her job. I, in turn, became anxious. To alleviate this problem, my doctor ordered a breast shield. Although it did draw the milk out, I felt awkward and out of place with a shield. Nobody else I knew had ever used one. I felt like a freak. Also, it took time to adjust the shield: I had to make sure that it was securely on my breast and that there was no air getting through. While I was trying to get all this straight, my baby was squirming and screaming for food. I was, and always felt that she was, uncomfortable. The shield was also a nuisance because when the baby sucked hard to get the milk, I felt as if she was going to pull the entire breast out. I was beginning to feel depressed — and, worse, resentful. This great natural thing called nursing was far from great or natural for me. I was starting to dread feeding times.

Another negative factor is that I felt compelled to nurse in private. I was embarrassed nursing in front of other people (except for my husband and mother) and believed that I was embarrassing them. Because of the nursing, I did not really want people to come and visit me. I was also ashamed of my enlarged breasts. I was not at all used to being big-bosomed.

Finally, I was simply sick of breast-feeding. For nine long months I had been carefully watching what I drank and ate, and now I was still forced to do so. I was worried if a glass of wine or a drink would hurt the baby, or if something I ate might cause her diarrhea or gas. I was tired of being limited in my time away from home, but no one else could feed our daughter. I was also worried about whether the baby was getting enough food and was satisfied. All I wanted to do was to be normal again, and to me that meant no longer nursing.

My last hurdle was the guilt, and that was the most difficult. I was not enjoying nursing, and friends and literature were all telling me that I was supposed to be enjoying it. Was something wrong with me? I was worried that if I stopped nursing I would be depriving my child of everything important — nutrition, warmth, and closeness. And then a friend of mine who is my age had to have a partial mastectomy. Here I was overflowing (literally) with milk, and she

48

was facing the traumatic experience of loss of a breast. The irony and unfairness of it all depressed me for weeks. Who was I to complain of my problems and frustrations about nursing when she had to have a breast removed?

I felt, too, that I had let my husband down a great deal. He had wanted me to nurse for two months. Since he rarely has asked anything major of me, I felt I should continue for his sake. When I told him of my decision to stop, he accepted my choice with his classic grace and kindness. But deep down, I sensed that I had greatly disappointed him.

Nursing is supposed to make you feel closer to your child. Because of my discomfort, guilt, and disappointments, it did not. I enjoyed my daughter much more and felt much closer to her once I was not nursing. I believe very strongly that a child, whatever age, senses negative feelings. I did not want to wind up with a fretful, nervous baby because of nursing.

My choice to give up nursing was a difficult one, and I worried afterward about whether I had made the right decision. My husband helped me to put the whole thing in its proper perspective when he said that I had made a choice that was right for me, which is what was important.

I certainly do not want to discourage mothers from nursing; however, I do think that it is important that mothers who, for whatever reasons, decide against breast-feeding should not be made to feel guilty or ashamed.

JOAN S. KLETZKER was in a supervisory position at a hospital before having a child. She plans to return to her work when her daughter is about a year old. The Kletzkers live in Glendale, Missouri.

Mothering a Late Weaner

SANDRA SHAPIRO FRIEDLAND

> *"Are the nummies workin'?"*
> *"I don't know. They might be empty."*
> *"I'll check," David announces, walking up to*
> *my chair and reaching under my shirt. His mouth*
> *is conveniently breast-high, and he begins to*
> *nurse while standing next to me.*
> *"Mmmmmmmmm," he sighs ecstatically, "the left*
> *one's full!"*

David will be three in a week. "Nummy" is his all-purpose word for my breasts, breast milk, and breast-feeding. Despite what he claims, I know that the "nummies" are almost dry, although the sweet trickle that remains is enough to remind him of his babyhood, comfort him when he's anxious, and lure him back for more — usually about once a day. Some days he forgets.

While I now accept the fact that my preschool-aged son still nurses, I did not always have such a liberal attitude about weaning. I instinctively *knew* I would breast-feed my babies, but I never imagined I would nurse a walking, talking child. During my first pregnancy, in fact, I was horrified by a three-foot-high suckling boy who nursed repeatedly while his mother led my introductory La Leche League meeting. The scene assaulted my pastel daydreams of nourishing my expected infant in rocking-chair seclusion.

These preconceptions faded during the twenty-one months I nursed David's older sister, Michelle. After I overcame engorgement, tender nipples, and the fear that I would smother her, breast-feeding was incredibly lovely. It seemed miraculous that *my breasts*, which had always embarrassed me, could be so useful and fulfilling. Nursing was the best I had to offer.

Rather than remove Michelle from the breast at some arbitrary age, I decided to let her continue nursing until she lost interest of her own accord. Her own development would determine when she would break away; I would not impose a separation on her. I saw it as the most natural — and least stressful — way for us to progress from a primarily physical relationship to a more verbal, interactive one.

Michelle's growth from nursing infant to nursing toddler was subtle and wonderful. Her behavior reinforced my opinions on weaning. She steadily reduced the time spent at the breast as she matured, eventually nursing only at dawn. One morning she simply asked for breakfast. Her independence, which came as a gentle surprise, brought both joy and sadness. Nursing an older baby had not been strange. Though unconventional and at times inconvenient, most often it was delightful. And so I looked forward to breast-feeding her sibling.

David arrived two-and-a-half years later, and I happily embarked on the same nursing course, aware that he could continue for several years but assuming he would follow Michelle's precedent. He did not. The longer he nursed, the more concerned I became about when he would stop. My faith in child-led weaning's benefits remains intact, but mothering a late weaner has not been easy. With the special rewards of nursing my son for such an extended period have come criticism, conflicts between my needs and David's, and doubts about my motivation for continuing to breast-feed.

Confident and content during David's first year, I offered him the breast whenever he cried, disregarding how long it had been since his last feeding. He required no supplements, and I delayed introducing solids and other liquids for six months. I could never bear to let him "cry it out" at night. If he awoke, my husband carried him to our bed where David peacefully nursed himself back to sleep. David thrived, and I enjoyed him. I credited our success, in large part, to breast-feeding and valued the intimacy it fostered. My husband praised my ability to nurture our children and agreed that allowing David to wean himself would promote his physical and psychological health.

Soon after David's first birthday, however, I began to sense pressure to wean him. I had received scant support for nursing Michelle once she no longer appeared infantile, but reactions to my nursing thirteen-month-old David were actually hostile. An older son at my breast was apparently more offensive than an older nursing daughter. Even though my husband still backed me, I felt compelled to examine my allegiance to child-led weaning.

Clearly, nursing David had evolved into more than a feeding method: it expressed my most basic love for my child and my instincts to care for him. Breast-feeding enabled me not only to satisfy his hunger and thirst, but also to allay his fears and insecurities, to soothe pain, and to assure him of consistent contact with me. David might want "nummy" twelve times, or twice, a day. Since he had no "regular" nursing times, the common technique of weaning by sequentially substituting a bottle or cup at regular meals did not fit our situation. And how could I — or any outsider — know precisely the right time to withdraw David's support system?

Child-led weaning seemed the logical extension of my actions and attitudes. Weaning David at fourteen months would have meant pushing him away, wearing clothing selected to defy his persistent fingers, and refusing his well-verbalized pleas. I believed such harsh measures to be unwarranted. The real issue for me was whether I would have the patience to wait until David developed his own ways to cope with physical and mental discomfort. I hoped that I could balance his requirements with mine.

This burgeoned into an Amazonian challenge. At fifteen months David was adorable but less complacent, quicker to anger, and more vulnerable than Michelle had been. Grabby and insistent about nursing, he hollered for "nummy" when I talked on the phone or entertained. At restaurants, grocery stores, and the swimming pool, he would reach inside my top or plaster his cheek on my bosom and cry. Still too young to reason with, he pounded his head or tore at my clothes when I didn't or couldn't comply with his wishes. If possible, I retreated with him to a car, rest room, or private place; otherwise, I nursed him wherever we happened to be, often in front of some shocked bystander who would mutter, "David, I didn't know you were *still* acting like a baby," or, "Don't you know that isn't good for him at his age?"

I resented David at times, and I felt guilty about it. I had taken a two-year leave of absence from teaching to care for him, but after sixteen months I grew impatient to return to work. I began tutoring three afternoons a week. These new absences unleashed additional demands to breast-feed — and more guilt. I escaped this trap by reserving time each day to read, work puzzles, or stroll with David. I tried to establish new activity patterns with him more like those he shared with his father.

Our parents and pediatrician asked how long I intended to nurse him. After eighteen months, I still answered "until he quits," despite their disapproval and my realization that no end was in sight. While David rarely stayed at the breast for long, his frequency hardly decreased. He didn't finger a blanket, suck his thumb, or treasure a toy; I was his huggy. I made every effort to be resourceful when he was upset — trying to distract him, rock him, or offer him a drink — but nursing remained the most effective pacifier. In some instances I was grateful that I *could* console him; at other times I longed for an alternative.

By twenty-one months, David began to understand that he occasionally had to wait for "nummy," and handling him became easier. He still showed no signs of weaning. My husband continued to be supportive, assuring me that David was merely maturing at a different rate than Michelle had. I could talk to few others. La Leche leaders shared my commitment to child-led weaning, yet their anecdotes and literature were too homey and oversimplified to answer my more intellectual questions — especially those concerning the psychological effects of a little boy's breast-feeding.

I wondered whether nursing stimulated David's oedipal fantasies. His two-year-old body language and speech were undeniably sexual. He liked to have his skin stroked and to stroke mine. He came to our bed and snuggled next to me. Frankly, his closeness felt good, but I chafed when he begged to "go to bed" with me, repeated how much he preferred "sleeping with Mommy" to his own bed, and insisted that my breast be fully removed from my clothing while he nursed. I began wearing prim nightshirts and disentangling his sleeping body from mine.

By day, David's desire to touch, cling, and climb corresponded to when I was busiest, most rushed, or craved privacy. Some confrontations were unavoidable, and I occasionally had to leave him screaming on the floor. If I took the time to nurse him, he would often suck once or twice and run away.

I asked myself about his self-image. He attended nursery school and never saw a classmate having "nummy." Did he feel different? He had learned not to nurse in front of others. Did he think he had something to hide? He would surely remember nursing. Would he resent it? My attitude, I reasoned, was crucial. Just as I took care not to humiliate Michelle, who still sucked her thumb and slept with a stuffed dog, so I had to be wary not to shame David. I suppressed any urge to tease or editorialize.

I searched in vain for reading on late weaning from the breast. Burton White's heralded *First Three Years of Life* alarmed me by reporting that, after eighteen months of age, a child spent "no time" seeking comfort. This statistic preposterously contradicted my experience. Fictional and biographical references to unweaned children often characterized a mother's instability, usually symbolizing her inadequate sex life, as in Toni Morrison's *Song of Solomon*. That novel flamed my fear that I was subconsciously prolonging David's breast-feeding stage because I liked the physical contact with him.

I watched for subtle reinforcements that might have encouraged him to seek the breast. For some time I had been cautious not to caress him while he nursed, which was not difficult at this stage since he wiped even a single uninvited kiss dramatically from his face. When he asked to breast-feed, I tried to be as matter-of-fact as possible. Yet there was no doubt that touching David — or Michelle — was wonderful. Some days I wanted to kiss him constantly and hug him until I ached. I tried to remember, however, that he was not my pet but an individual with distinct desires. He could be deliciously affectionate on his own terms: he determined our "cuddle times" just as he did our breast-feeding schedule.

Perhaps I was artificially extending David's dependency because he completed our two-child family. I loved being pregnant, giving birth, and, of course, nursing. Facing my life without a childbearing future was a depressing prospect, but I realized that I couldn't use David to fill that anticipated void. I resisted the temptation to call him "Baby" or to talk to him like one. I did not harange him to be a "big boy," but my nonverbal behavior clearly dictated unbabylike responses. Meanwhile I compulsively took pictures, recorded his voice, and wrote about him. It was as if I were trying to suspend time so I could work through my painful transition from life-giver to life-guider.

———————

At David's two-and-a-half-year checkup, my pediatrician said that David nursed to control me and that I must win the battle. Her warnings increased my self-doubts. I panicked. Maybe his nursing *had* gotten out of hand. He might never give up something he enjoyed so much. If I stopped nursing him abruptly, his development might suffer. Were I to continue, my negative feelings would be obvious to him. I had to resolve my uncertainty.

I talked to my husband and watched our son. David acted happy and free-spirited. Our wills did clash, although not more often than one might expect with a bright, assertive child. In addition, I felt reasonably in charge of my own routine, which included a part-time job, exercise, and time for myself and the rest of my family. I perceived David's nursing not as a means of control but as his method of dealing with situations and sensations he could not manage otherwise. As his need to nurse diminished daily, while his internal resources multiplied, I grew calmer.

I did impose my preference in one area: nighttime nursing. He could still come to our bed if he awoke, but he could not have "nummy" while it was dark. We experienced two terrible nights. He cried to nurse and I held him, hoping to reassure, not frustrate him. On the third night he slipped into our bed and quietly went back to sleep. He displayed no signs of increased tension during the day, bolstering my confidence.

No longer nursing at night, he began skipping some days. By thirty-four months he was toilet-trained, attended day camp, slept at his grandmother's, and roamed with the neighborhood gang. We were so pleased with his progress, in fact, that my husband and I planned our first trip by ourselves since his birth. Leaving him, however, proved complicated. I impulsively called his school to warn his teachers to expect a change. The closer our departure date drew, the more instruction lists I left for the sitter. I didn't know whether my absence would cause David to stop breast-feeding, and felt I was betraying my hard-won principles of child-led weaning. I cried all the way to the airport. Once I was physically away, my composure returned, and I enjoyed our travels and relished the time alone with my husband. Yet whenever I passed a baby, I caught myself checking my breasts to see if they were full.

David managed extremely well during our ten-day separation. He seemed inches taller and surprisingly mature when I returned. Within hours of our homecoming, though, he shyly asked to nurse. I welcomed the chance to assuage my guilt about going away before he had weaned, although I half expected that his successful experience without nursing would enable him to abandon it. Apparently neither of us was quite prepared to do so.

Two months later, as we plan his birthday party, he informs me that three-year-olds don't have "nummy." I know he is right. I watch him trying to separate from me; his conflicting drives to be grown-up and to remain a baby are powerful and poignant. After a long struggle, I have gained perspective on his nursing. I don't blame his occasional misbehavior or my periodic irritation at his possessiveness solely on his unweaned status. I recognize that his slow parting with breast-feeding has been just one aspect of his growth toward self-sufficiency, a goal he approaches at his own pace.

Author's Postscript

David weaned himself soon after his third birthday. Ironically, when I realized he hadn't nursed for several days, I could not remember the final time. After about a week, a teasing tone in his voice, he asked for "nummy" again. With surprising ease I told him honestly that he no longer needed to nurse, and he accepted my response. He repeated his request a few times in the days that followed; my answer remained consistent and he never pressed me. Then it was over. Deeply absorbed in a writing project, I didn't allow myself to dwell on David's passage from my last baby to my youngest child. I marveled at how well both of us had managed the transition.

Two months later, however, he saw a younger cousin nursing. For several days David whined for "nummy" and finally asked for a bottle, something he had rarely done. He looked pathetic clutching his Even Flo, but I did not want to nurse him. I missed the warmth, convenience, and simplicity of breast-feeding, but we had learned new ways to relate to one another. After extra cuddling and some priceless talk about the "good old nummy days," he regained his former confidence and independence.

Now, four months since David has stopped nursing, my breasts look small and flaccid. Last night in the shower I checked to see whether any milk remained. Several creamy drops splashed down my body, mixing with warm water and sudden tears.

SANDRA SHAPIRO FRIEDLAND considered "when, not whether, to have children." Both her children were born Lamaze-style, and she returned to work as a high school English teacher when each child was two years old. A resident of Westfield, New Jersey, Sandra has taken a year off to write.

4

Staying Home

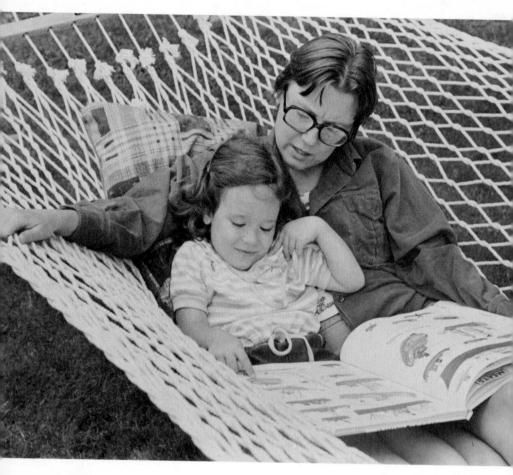

Joan Albert

Staying Home and Liking It

EMILY L. TIPERMAS

A few years back, had I peered into a crystal ball and seen that I was to become the unemployed mother of a toddler, I would have sunk into the blackest of depressions. The toddler, I would have been thrilled about; it's the unemployed part that would have thrown me.

In those days, it was incomprehensible to me why any woman would actually choose to stay at home with small children. I did, to be sure, know a few "full-time" mothers who were doing creative, worthwhile things with the relative freedom afforded to them by not being rigorously bound to a nine-to-five regime. But the majority of mothers I casually observed were, in my view, mired in mindless activity. It was beyond me how they could obligingly sacrifice years to sit home and cater to the whims and tantrums of the preschool set. Their tales of boredom, frustration, and craziness made me cringe. I indeed wanted children, but saw no problem with placing them in the care of highly competent baby sitters. Moreover, I was assured by several women who were doing precisely this that it caused no discernible damage to their kids, and that was all I needed to hear. If they could successfully juggle a career and family, thanks to quality day care, there was no earthly reason why I should be unable to do the same.

The speed with which this conviction began to crumble following confirmation of my pregnancy can only be attributed to the overwhelming difference between my concerns for a hypothetical child and the emotions I was now experiencing for the tiny being growing within me. In the throes of budding maternal devotion, I was finding it impossible to sustain the original zeal about leaving my flesh and blood each day in the charge of hired help. While it had all seemed so logical, manageable, and acceptable when initially thought out, I was suddenly registering mild panic about potentially negative consequences of substitute mothering.

Yet I could hardly disregard the other side of the coin. I had recently received a master's degree, and I wanted a shot at the job opportunities that would probably open up to me. After all, I had not sweated through countless papers and exams for nothing.

As an attempt to extricate myself from this dilemma, I began to read all I could about babies, early child development, and parenting. It quickly became apparent that there was no golden answer. Some authors argued that children can endure the continual absence of a mother with no ill effects. Others maintained that in the long run a sizable crop of personal disorders could be anticipated. What was I to do? Although I could interpret any insistence of the superiority of round-the-clock parent care as little more than a traditional contrivance used to keep women in their place, for me personally it nevertheless posed a cause for serious consideration.

During this period I happened to meet a woman who was just returning to work, after taking off the previous six months to give birth and attend to her infant son. He presently was being cared for by a sitter who came to her home daily. When I inquired how things were going for her, she responded with a chuckle, *"He's* adjusting." I recall chuckling along with her, but when I later thought about her remark, it lacked its prior hilarity. Having read about separation anxiety and attachment behavior, all I could envision was a confused, frightened, and thoroughly miserable infant being forced to deal maturely with a bewildering situation. I tried to imagine how I would react to going off each morning against a backdrop of wails: would I feel relief and liberation to be out of the house or debilitating apprehension? Did I honestly possess the capacity to handle regular farewell hysteria?

Coming down the stretch of the final trimester, I concluded that it was best to play it by ear. That I wanted eventually to return to the working realm was beyond dispute, but setting an absolute date for departure was out of the question. My confusion at that point really necessitated a testing of the waters of motherhood before I could make any kind of rational decision. My husband wasn't pressuring me in either direction; he shared the same uneasiness I did about the wisdom of leaving a baby to spend the bulk of its waking hours in the care of an outsider, yet he also sympathized with my needs for career gratification. In short, he was prepared to support whatever position I took.

On my last day of work — and three weeks before my due date

— labor began. Twenty-four hours later, Suzannah emerged into the world. I wouldn't go so far as to say that the moment I held her all job aspirations vanished, but whether because of the unique exhilaration of producing life, the novelty of a first child, or hormones, I was certainly more enthralled with this marvelous little creature than I was with anything else, including a career.

That kind of euphoria, however, can be quickly dissolved by the endurance test of the early weeks under the same roof with a newborn. Love can conquer a lot, but it can't diminish the physical duress and interminable exhaustion of days and weeks without adequate rest. More than once I was driven to scream, "I can't take it anymore," and throughout the agonizing wait for Suzannah to achieve a civilized eating and sleeping schedule, I often doubted that I would ever again feel like a sane human being. With life taking on the semblance of one endless succession of feedings, diaperings, rockings, burpings, and spit-ups, the prospect of going back to work looked appealing beyond words; all I craved was the strength to find myself a job, and to get there each day.

It's hard to say when the craving stopped. The prospect of working never really lost its appeal, but I was slowly coming to realize that as much as I believed that career-minded women should not be harnessed to their children at the expense of their goals, I had to admit that I did not feel right about leaving Suzannah.

I listened to rave reviews about various day-care sitters, and I had no doubt that there truly existed sitters who merited such acclaim. But for every wonderful Mary, I also heard about the undependable Bessie who showed up late in the morning or sometimes not at all. This same Bessie would perform her duties with stunning negligence, and then one day announce that she was resigning, leaving in her wake a distraught child lacking the grown-up emotional and intellectual mechanisms to cope with abrupt desertion and the arrival of yet another caretaker. Perhaps I was the victim of excessive anxiety, but frankly the possibility that this could actually occur — despite the most rigorous of screenings — was instrumental in destroying the attraction of a salaried fill-in parent.

In addition to my apprehension about day care, I was also not convinced that anyone would give attention to Suzannah's development and emotional needs as readily, tenderly, lovingly, and sympathetically as I assuredly would. On top of that, I did not relish subjecting my daughter to a situation less than perfect while she was still incapable of articulating a complaint. After all, how would I know what went on the moment I disappeared out the door? Would the seemingly kind, motherly employee sit glued to the television set for hours on end while my child languished in a playpen? Would she be a subscriber to the "cry-it-out" theory, which ran completely counter to my own approach? Would she have weird notions of discipline that I would have had no opportunity to notice when I was present? Suzannah certainly couldn't tell me.

At least once a day I took Suzannah out to a store, a friend's, a museum, a library, a park, or an exercise class designed especially for babies her age. In our own home, she and I entertained a stream of visitors. When comparing this type of exposure and stimulation to the repetitious routine she would have in day care, I was again unable to muster much enthusiasm for the latter.

As for Suzannah's emotional equilibrium, as long as I was in close proximity, she was basically content, outgoing, uninhibited, and relaxed; when I walked off, the tears would rapidly descend. This behavior was typical and predictable, but when I contemplated constantly thrusting Suzannah into an arrangement that could provoke it — specifically, a world devoid of the security of my presence — job hunting fell to a very low priority.

I may be creating the impression that my hesitancy to rejoin the working ranks rested solely on a preoccupation with the hazards of day care. Actually there was another factor with which I had never bargained: the effect of Suzannah's disruptive sleep performance on my level of energy. Unlike those ideal children who ease themselves into a normal bedtime pattern after a few torturous weeks, Suzannah failed to give in until she was two months old. And then, after gracing us with twelve uninterrupted hours in the sack for the next three months, she broke her streak at the five-month mark. From that point on through her thirteenth month she awoke religiously every night, anywhere between one and three, with ear-splitting screams, until a beverage was produced. The inevitable result of this — for someone who requires eight consecutive hours of sleep — was awesome fatigue every morning. How, I thought, could I ever jump up, rush out to a job, and handle it with any shred of competence, feeling as wiped out as I did? In a burst of self-discovery, I recognized that, as luck would have it, I was neither Wonderwoman nor Supermom.

It has now been a year and a half that I've been full-timing it with Suzannah, and I harbor no regrets about what I've done. She's developing beautifully, and whether or not this can be credited to genes, my input, or a combination of both, I deem this in and of itself worth the time and effort I've devoted to her. As for the deferment of my career plans, I don't think a year and a half or longer is necessarily going to have much influence upon my future in the grander scheme of things. Indeed, if a career were my single objective or interest in life, I would probably have opted not to have had children at all. I cannot deny that I occasionally wonder if in fact my undivided attentions have really made a substantial difference in Suzannah — whether "quality time" in smaller dose might not have been just as effective. Perhaps, but I would always have had misgivings if I had turned her over to day care.

When it comes right down to it, I have to confess that I'm getting a genuine kick out of the whole child-rearing process. I don't mean to say that each minute of every day has been a memorable, delightful experience. On the contrary, annoyance, anger, aggravation, and weariness are sprinkled through a normal week. But to counteract this, there is immense fascination, excitement, humor, and, yes, fulfillment in the process of assisting and witnessing my child surge through the web of growth phases.

I often speak with other women who have also chosen to set aside career strivings temporarily for the sake of children. As in my case, they have neither been browbeaten into mothering nor are they adherents of the notion that child care is "woman's work." Rather, their decisions have evolved from much intensive thought, debate, and personal soul-searching. What I've gathered from them is that I haven't been alone in finding it difficult to follow my instincts and resolve to remain at home with a baby in a climate that frequently greets such a move with pure condescension. When you sense that others perceive you as having caved in to a traditional role — that you are doing nothing particularly noteworthy or commendable — it's hard not to feel anything but insulted and defensive.

A friend of mine told me that at a party she and her husband attended after her son was born, a woman came up to her and, after introductions, asked what sort of work she did. My friend, sick and tired of her propensity to downplay child care and dwell upon past accomplishments to elicit appropriate respect, flatly stated, "I stay home and take care of my baby." The woman smiled feebly and excused herself to move on. My friend felt as though she had just been given the official stamp of disapproval. Unfortunately, incidents similar to this are all too commonplace and help make the already burdensome choice to stay home even tougher.

I have every intention of going back to work eventually, but I must first feel confident that I'm getting Suzannah off to the best possible start in life. This is as important to me as my own pursuits, and so I unequivocally place child care on a par with a career. In the final analysis, how other mothers approach the career-versus-motherhood conflict is of little relevance to me because they may be operating under different conditions and with different values. I have simply done what I believe to be necessary and have restructured my career dreams around my decision. And, so far, so good.

With a thirtieth birthday staring her in the face, EMILY L. TIPER-MAS concluded that the time was ripe to plunge into motherhood. She lives outside of Washington, D.C., and hopes to rejoin the salaried force part-time in the near future.

The Artist as Mother

SU-LI HUNG

For as long as I can remember I never really considered myself one who would become another traditional Chinese woman, like my grandmother and my mother. There, generation after generation of

66

women have taken care of their homes, helping their husbands and raising their children. In this unchanging way, the whole life of a woman passes within the small world of the family.

I felt that my art work and the study of literature would suit me much more than a life of staying home, bearing children, cooking good food, and having a model home.

Originally I thought that I would never have to change this way of thinking. But after five years of marriage, Richard — who is also an artist — and I decided to have a child. I found that I could no longer maintain my original ideas. Even though I had my own ambitions, I could not resist the desire to have a soft baby and a warm house. So I had Benji, with his head full of black hair and his face wrinkled like an old man's, sucking eagerly at my breast. And what a great feeling it was to be a mother!

At that time, we lived in a ninth-floor loft with windows on three sides, which let in luxuriant sunlight and looked out on the most fantastic views of New York City. The Manhattan Bridge was just outside our window. Day and night the traffic sped by. The East River had freighters and small tugboats and flocks of seagulls. The Empire State Building glowed beautifully at night to the north. To the west, the twin towers of the World Trade Center pointed up into the sky like two gigantic fingers. Richard and I loved, lived, and worked in this studio for three-and-a-half years before Benji was born. We had great hopes for the work we were doing there.

Unfortunately, this ideal loft for artists was most unsuitable as a nursery. In the summer the black smoke from the smokestack, which came from Brooklyn across the East River, was carried by the wind through our open windows. In no time at all, the baby's blanket had a sprinkling of black soot. The building's elevator man was poorly paid and often found excuses to slip away to drink with his friends. From our top floor loft, we would have to carry the heavy baby carriage up and down nine flights, passing the noisy and congested floors of the dress-making factories, to do our shopping, laundry, and other errands. Benji and I would try to stay at home as much as possible to avoid that unpleasant journey, and gradually became almost prisoners in our loft.

But the most difficult time was the winter. Heat was available only during the factories' working hours, eight to four. And there was never enough heat to reach the ninth floor. At night, when I was nursing Benji, it was almost as cold inside as the snowy world outside. I wrapped the baby in three blankets, but we both still shivered in the freezing air.

Richard and I were not so dramatic as to throw our paintings into a fire to keep us warm (as movies sometimes show artists doing), but I could not help thinking that our way of life was not right for Benji. I even doubted the wisdom of having had a child. I wondered how I could go on in this fashion.

I still remember the first few months after his birth, when I would wake suddenly in the middle of the night, full of alarm, and rush to his bedside to make sure that he was still there and still breathing; he looked so delicate and so vulnerable. This kind of imagination and worry drove me to the point of exhaustion, making it difficult to experience the full joy of motherhood.

For one as totally unconscious of practical matters as I, trying to cope with wifely chores such as cleaning, sewing, and taking care of the baby was difficult. I wanted to give Benji all my love and attention, but I was also much annoyed by the petty details of the household. I begrudged the time spent not painting, reading, or thinking. On the one hand, I would enjoy the warmth I experienced in breast-feeding my son, hearing his gurgles, and wiping his soft baby down. On the other hand, in my mind I was vacantly casting about for inspiration. For a long time, I had been completely cut off from movies, museums, and jazz clubs. Once when one of my Chinese friends, here in New York, sent me all the books, magazines, and newspapers he had read over the past few months, I was close to tears. These Chinese publications, almost impossible for me to get, were like food for my soul.

While I was concentrating on being a good mother, I found myself isolated from the outside world. I saw very little of my friends because I was so absorbed in my baby. He was the main topic of my conversation, and my childless friends felt that a baby was like a pet; they could not sympathize with either my excitement or my frustration. I was stuck in the routine of my narrow world.

Finally I took up my brush and started to draw Benji when he was sleeping, when he was gurgling to himself, and when he first discovered — to his delight — that the things moving about were arms and legs which belonged to him. I tried to capture the feelings of these moments, the utter simplicity of that beauty.

After Benji turned six months, Richard could take care of him without needing me there. I could go out to draw, find subjects, see friends, close the door to read by myself, and write. Especially at night, after the baby slept, I would work more intensely because time was so precious. I felt so happy knowing that even without my constant presence my baby was being well taken care of by his father. With Richard helping me, and with Benji becoming more independent, my art work gradually became central to my life again. I combined my work and parenthood by doing sketches of him and his friends playing, eventually making them into woodcuts. I was not the full-time artist I used to be, but I was again an artist — and that was enough.

My son is now almost two and a half. The frustration of the past years of infancy is behind me. I find it marvelous now to watch him grow. Like a splendid work of art, each day he shows me a new side of himself. Art is creative, and so in its way is play. I discover in playing with Benji that our purposes are not so different: we both seek happiness and beauty.

SU-LI HUNG was born in Taiwan, where she remained until she completed college. She met her husband at the Art Students' League in New York City. The Sloats lived in Taiwan, where Benji's first language was Chinese. Now back in New York, Benji is — without any difficulty — bilingual.

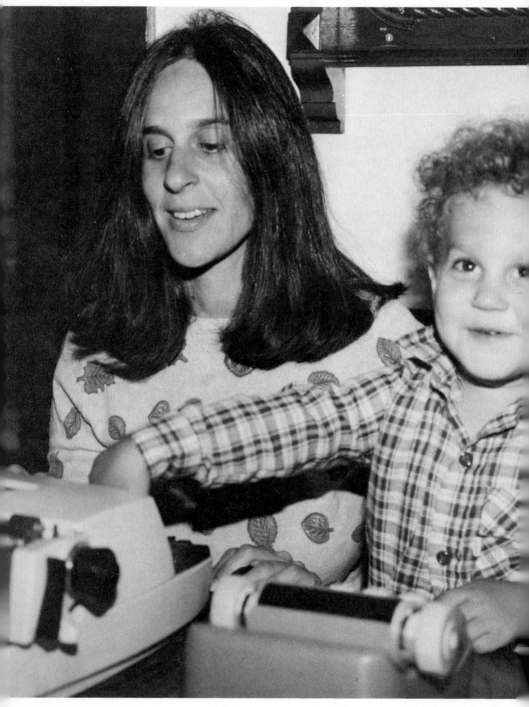

Daniel E. Little

Redefining Work

ELLEN A. ROSEN

*I like what is in the work — the chance to find
yourself.
Your own reality — for yourself, not for others.*
— Joseph Conrad, *Heart of Darkness*

When I stopped working at the end of my first pregnancy, I had a wait-and-see attitude about returning to my job. As Rebecca grew, I found the prospect of continuing to work as a social worker less compelling than the possibilities for fulfilling work as a homemaker and mother. I believe this is partially explained by the fact that both my job and my family required me to nurture. Once my need to "mother" was satisfied at home, I was less drawn to a job where nurturing was a primary requirement and satisfaction.

Since leaving that job, I have tried to redefine my concept of work — placing less emphasis on making money, social status, and professional recognition — so that I can apply it to my current life as a mother and a homemaker. Although I am convinced most of the time that mothering and homemaking are, in fact, "work," I am less confident of how others view my job. I am uncomfortable when I tell someone I have just met that I do not work outside my home. I even feel uneasy as I write this and apply the word *work* to my current life. Still, over time, I have become increasingly persuaded of the value and importance of what I do because of my experience as a mother.

Motherhood is my work because it is a challenge and a commitment with opportunities both for self-expression and for developing and testing my inner resources. It is also my work because I have become skilled and competent at it. Applying my energies toward creating a comfortable lifestyle for my family and me has been both a struggle and an adventure, and has surprised me in its capacity to engage my attention, enrich my life, and change me.

Before I had my own family, my contact with younger children was mostly limited to infrequent gatherings of my extended family. I neither baby-sat as an adolescent nor felt especially comfortable

71

with children. Still, the idea of having my own children appealed to me. I was not sure what to expect from them, or how I would feel about sharing my life with them, and the strong pleasure that I now take in mothering my children was unexpected.

My daughters have enhanced my life in many ways. I appreciate the sense of self-renewal they have created for me as we deal together with different developmental issues and life experiences. As a parenting adult, I feel an obligation to revisit my past in order to use it effectively for my children.

The longing for a dog I had felt as a five-year-old was at last satisfied eight years ago, when Una came to live with us. The playful, caring relationship that Rebecca, age six, and Molly, age three, have with Una pleases me as their mother, but also fulfills an unmet wish from my own childhood.

The acuity of my daughters' responses to the passage of time, captured in events like holiday celebrations and seasonal changes, makes me feel grounded in both change and continuity. I encourage their delight in these yearly highlights because I too am sustained by ceremony and the rhythms of nature.

We have a special drawer for ritual objects like the Chanukah menorah and birthday games. This year, as we put away the menorah, Rebecca asked, "What's next?" We discussed the fact that Valentine's Day was coming soon. That night, as I walked past her room, I saw Rebecca carefully examining her valentines from last year. Recently, as it started to snow, Rebecca asked, "When's spring?" A few minutes later, she began to recall last winter when our friend, who had come for Friday night dinner, stayed for the whole weekend during a paralyzing snowstorm. The easy convergence of anticipation and reminiscence in my daughters' viewpoints connects past, present, and future time for me and adds depth and dimension to my life.

───────────

I am sometimes profoundly touched by my daughters. These heightened feelings happen publicly and privately, at formal and ordinary moments, as I observe my children and interact with them. At her school assembly, for example, I watched Rebecca participate in her class program with pride and pleasure; and recently, as I tucked Molly in bed while she slept, she awakened and told me, for the first time, about her seven imaginary friends. These joyous but ephemeral moments are memorable and bonding.

My daughters are lively, stimulating companions who know that I enjoy their company. Their trust in me, and my comfort with them, frees me from self-conscious feelings I have in other relationships. With my children, I have a singular opportunity to express my feelings directly and to be playful. The absolute nature of our bond contributes to an atmosphere of honesty and spontaneity that is expressed both physically and verbally.

When we walk to the library early on a sunny morning and feel exuberant together, I can tousle their hair and hug them. On the other hand, when I am angry with them, I am able to say, "You are getting on my nerves." When we need to "let off steam," we can dance to the music on the radio or wrestle on the mattress on the hall floor. At other times, we sing extemporaneous songs or speak gibberish to each other.

My daughters enlighten me about myself. Their presence acts as a constant, ever-changing reflection of me as well as a source of feedback, as I see myself mirrored in their mannerisms, attitudes, and relationships. Sometimes the image I see is kaleidoscopic, and pleases me. When Rebecca or Molly chats with a dog or a cat, I am happy because I hear a confirmation of my own sense of whimsy. At other times, the image appears as in a distorted mirror, and disturbs me. Early in the school year, Robert and I spoke with Rebecca's teacher, who felt that Rebecca was trying too hard to please her and was excessively sensitive to her criticism of Rebecca's work. While the situation has improved, it caused me to consider my high expectations of myself and my own difficulties in handling criticisms, and what, if any, impact these qualities of mine had on Rebecca's school situation.

The process of learning to handle the intense interpersonal fluctuations in day-to-day life with my daughters over the last six years has changed me. Recently, we had a prolonged siege of illness in our family. Within a five-week period, Molly had chicken pox and two ear infections, and Rebecca had chicken pox. Since my children were born, this was the longest time that I have been at home nursing and caring for them. I was worn out by interrupted sleep and frustrated because I was giving more to my children while receiving fewer "rewards." My daughters were less interesting and less affectionate than usual. My confinement upset me — I was less in control of my time, and while I was concerned about my children's well-being, I was equally concerned about the effects of their illnesses on my own life. At first I felt remorseful that I was concerned for us equally. Once I acknowledged this and decided to salvage the time that I was at home, I was able to become more flexible and less resentful. The children and I made bread, and I tackled some correspondence and sewing that needed attention.

I remember when Rebecca was sick as an infant and how difficult it was for me then to cope with the demands of illness, the disruption of sleep, time, and plans, and the disappointment of unequal return for my attention and care. I also remember that I felt more passive and immobilized when she was sick as an infant than I had when she was sick recently. My ability to be more adaptable in difficult circumstances was a direct result of my learning, as a mother, to deal with restrictive situations over which I had little control.

———————

While the expansion of my life from parents' daughter to daughters' mother, from child to parent, has placed limitations on my freedom, it has also allowed me to mature. Accepting responsibility for my daughters' development, committing myself to the time and effort involved in doing this work conscientiously, and discovering deep satisfaction in the process have brought me a sense of personal extension beyond myself, a propelling connectedness through time and space, to other mothers — past, present, and future — who are also responsible for the maintenance of daily life. These developments in my life have also brought me a deepening concern for the future of the human community. My value system has necessarily become more clearly articulated as I decide how to use my free time, as well as what personal beliefs and attitudes I want to share with my daughters. Nurturing my children and serving as a role model for them have made me feel like a more fully developed human being. I have examined my capacities for perception, thought, feeling, and action on my children's behalf and have felt these powers ripen in the process.

In relation to my children, I see my work as a "witness" and

a "shaper"* — observing and influencing their emerging consciousness and sensibilities. I watch and listen to my daughters, then try
to translate what I believe to be their interests and concerns into
appropriate stimulation and support. This work is validated by Rebecca and Molly themselves and by their positive development. I
have learned that I am most helpful to my daughters when I am
clear about my own responses to people and situations. When I can
recognize my own reactions, it is easier for me to respond to their
needs instead of my own. In this way, I find motherhood an opportunity for increasing my self-awareness.

When Rebecca was a toddler, we attended a parent-child "tot-
lot" at a local community center. Rebecca sometimes spent the
entire two-hour playtime standing at my side and watching the
other children. Because of her behavior, I felt ill at ease, as though
her quiet assessments reflected on my mothering. Once I realized
that I wanted her to interact with the other children in order to
make me feel more comfortable, I was able to allow her to deal
with this situation according to her own style. We continued to
attend "tot-lot," and Rebecca continued to observe. Today, at six,
she has friends and plays well with her peers.

Much of my time is spent working toward a richly textured life for
my family, where the quality of our life and times together is a high
priority. I strive to create a common family identity by chronicling
our lives in photo albums, films, or children's art portfolios. Having
an organized but lively household — full of friends and family,
animals, music, and projects — is important as we work in these
early years to create patterns and foundations for the years to come.

One advantage to considering my family as my work is that
it enables me to devote my free time to myself. Where mothers
with outside occupations feel they must devote their time off to
their children, I have felt comfortable using my time to pursue
ongoing projects or develop personal interests.

* In *Grendel*, John Gardner's retelling of the Beowulf legend from the monster's viewpoint, the "shaper" is the harpist-singer who uses "the givens of his time
and place and tongue . . . spins it all together with harp runs and hoots" and makes
his listeners think that "what they think is alive."

There is a strong counterpoint to everything I have previously written that colors many of my upbeat feelings about the last six years. It is composed of the doubts, fears, and concerns I have about my decision to stay at home, particularly its implications for my future. One aspect of my ambivalence relates to my husband. I compare the settings in which we both work — the downtown business and financial community versus the self-supervised world of our home. To the extent that the high-powered atmosphere of my husband's world appeals to me, I am jealous; to the extent that it repels me, I feel spared, sheltered, and protected from it. Because I make only a negligible financial contribution to our lifestyle, I have sometimes felt my authority diminished in joint decision making. Sometimes this seems to result from Robert's condescending attitude toward me and, at other times, from my own feelings of inequality. Finally, I feel uncomfortable that the chance to use these early years of motherhood as an opportunity, not only a restriction, is possible because I am supported by a man at whose "expense" my growth occurred. I believe that Robert would appreciate the chance to be free from the financial pressures of earning a living, as I have been, in order to explore his own interests.

Then, too, I have troubling feelings about myself in relation to other women. I am bothered by a sense of privilege because I have not had to work. When I compare myself to women who must support themselves, my sense of relief at staying home out of the "real world" changes to a sense of isolation and an elitist exemption from the "realities" of life. Also, I tend to think of myself as less capable than mothers who not only work at home as I do, but who also have outside occupations.

Although I foresee that my new work will derive from interests I have developed and pursued while at home, I still wonder if I will be penalized for my choice and whether future full-time reentry into the job market will be more difficult because I have stayed at home.

Regardless, these years have represented a welcome time off. Since I find that my daughters now require less time and energy than before, I look forward to filling some space in my life. I have grown and changed because of my experience with my children, and am satisfied by my sense of having done a good job with them and my household. As I now face the prospect of doing new and different work, I am glad that I spent the last six years as I did.

ELLEN A. ROSEN and her family live in a Victorian three-flat, which they renovated, in Chicago.

Mothering Others, Mothering My Own

SELMA DENDY

Several years ago I became the first young mother in my group of friends to be divorced. Things were different then, both in the world and in me — I was inexperienced, and I felt an overwhelming sense of guilt about what I was "doing" to my one-year-old son and four-year-old daughter.

To provide an income and built-in friends for my kids, I started a family day-care group in my home. My guilt over being a single parent and having to leave my children wouldn't allow me to go back to my prematernal job as a junior high art teacher. I have continued to do day care at home, because I am good at this job, because my children need me at home — and also because some still-lingering sense of guilt prevents me from working outside my home. Ironically, of course, I deal every day with mothers who *do* leave their young children to work outside the home. Some of these children are in day care all day, five days a week: some are infants only a few weeks old when they begin care. Frankly, I couldn't have done that with my own children.

Occasionally I must deal with feelings of resentment and jealousy: these women are going out into the "real world," the adult world, while I am "home with the kids." Nor does it matter that I am my own boss, a child-care professional, consultant, master's degree recipient, and supporter of two children.

77

Sometimes I find myself passing judgment on these mothers: they are leaving babies who need them. Of course I am aware that it is because of my care and concern that these women feel comfortable in going off to work each day, to careers that are *their* specialty, just as child care is mine. I know too that it is not easy for them to leave their children. It is not unusual for one or another of them to drop off her child in the morning and leave my home with tear-filled eyes. Still, I sometimes wonder how they can do it.

Basically, I'm very happy with my job. I am good at working with children, and I know it. Ironically, though, I have a hard time mothering my own. Why do I "mother" other women's children with calmness, competence, love, and even joy, yet allow my own kids to get to me so easily?

My day-care children might be with me for three or four years at most, but Pam and Davey are a lifetime commitment. My day-care children go home at five o'clock. My own kids do not. Also, Pam and David are now older than the day-care children — and therefore better able to argue, cajole, and manipulate.

I don't really question my mothering skills or judgment, unless they are affected by the stronger and deeper emotions that motherhood engenders. All the developmental hurdles — moving from bottle to cup, giving up the pacifier, becoming toilet-trained, eating a variety of foods, learning to cooperate, accepting discipline — are relatively easy to accomplish in day care, because these are not my own children. We are not engaged in a life-or-death power struggle, which I believe mothering entails. Because I'm not their mother, they don't have to relinquish any power to me in the process of toilet-training, nor do I "win" anything. It is just my job. I know that eventually they'll accomplish their tasks, and I'm not as completely invested in the outcome. But for some reason this is not true with my own children: I don't have that certainty that the right things will come to pass.

I remember myself as a new mother and my feelings of total inadequacy as I consulted Dr. Spock about toilet-training. I would hold my breath when I put Pamie on the potty seat, and feel depressed and helpless when she would have what I was sure were deliberate "accidents." My whole emotional life and sense of self-worth seemed to hang in the balance of her success with toilet-training.

It is interesting how much more easily David toilet-trained, just a couple of years later, when he was part of my day-care group. He had the advantage of being a part of a group, and subject to group dynamics and peer-group influence. And I was so busy with the group as a whole that I had very limited time to "power struggle" with him about it, or even to focus on it for that matter. Our struggles resumed, of course, as soon as Davey outgrew the group.

Day-care discipline? That's easy: a few minutes of isolation on the "Big Chair." But disciplining my own kids is not nearly as easy or clear-cut. In fact, Pam and David once accused me of loving the day-care children more, "because you never spank *them*." As I tried to explain that I have a different role with them, I felt both sad and amused.

As my day-care mothers watch me effectively dealing with a herd of their little children, they seem to feel that I have all the answers. I don't. And I'm not always a very good mother. I probably have had the same problems with my kids that my day-care parents have at home with theirs, the very same children who respond so well in the day-care setting. The simple reason that I'm so effective in day care is that I'm less emotionally involved.

I love Pam and Davey deeply, but often I would rather be dealing with my day-care group: it's so much easier. The day-care children actually listen to me; they don"t continually challenge or assault me with their needs and arguments. It's easier to tickle tiny feet while changing a diaper than to justify to thirteen-year-old Pam why she can't watch "Charlie's Angels."

To my day-care children I'm a loving authority figure, and they accept my authority. But it is Pam and Davey's task to challenge me, to engage me in power struggles, to break away.

My children and I both feel and express more extreme negative and positive feelings toward each other than my day-care children and I do. Although this intensity makes things more complicated, it is also much more rewarding. Years ago, the idea that I could love my kids but not always like them would have horrified the idealistic side of me. By now I've grown used to it.

Born in New York City, SELMA DENDY is registered to have six children in a family day-care setting by the Massachusetts Office for Children. The age range of her group is infancy through four.

5

Going to Work

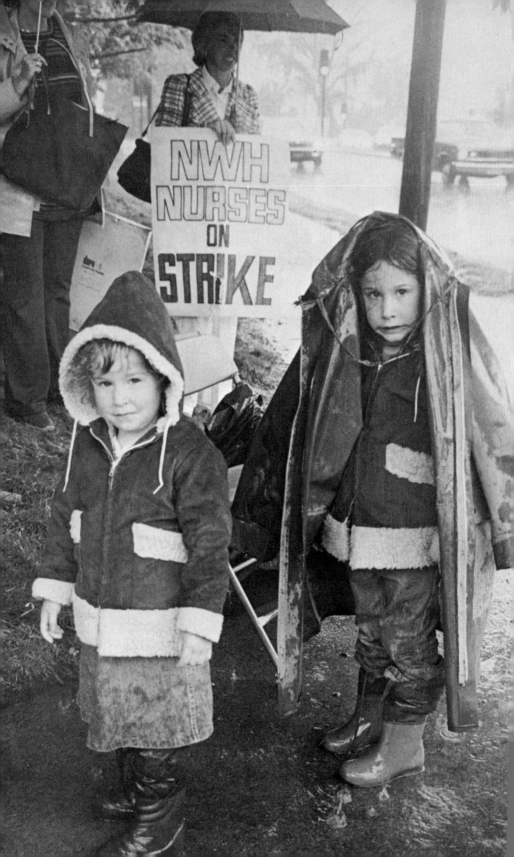

One Year Home Was Enough

MADELINE ETTIN ISRAEL

I grew up in a Bronx neighborhood noted for apartment buildings, corner stores, the New York Yankees, and families in which mothers did not work. This was so accepted that the public schools, right through junior high, sent pupils home for lunch, confident that they would be met by nourishing food and maternal comfort. In my house, I was greeted by a hot lunch (no peanut butter and jelly for me), my mother, and often my grandmother, who would listen to my stories, make sure that I finished my lunch, and send me back to school. A classmate whose mother returned to work was the object of universal pity. Not until high school did I meet people whose mothers worked, but they were from the more exotic Manhattan. Few of my friends had mothers who worked, and *none* had mothers who were out of the home before their children were of school age.

From as early as I can remember, perhaps because I sensed maternal dissatisfaction, perhaps because I sensed there was another world beyond the confines of my Bronx neighborhood, I did not want to be a "housewife." I felt uneasy with the notion of children being the center of one's life, wanted a career, and was not at all convinced that motherhood and I were compatible. To me, motherhood was synonymous with housewives, station wagons, and staying at home, all the things that I wanted to reject.

Married for five years, working at an interesting and challenging job, with good friends and a full life, I turned thirty. I began (perhaps irrationally) to fear that my childbearing years were coming to an end and that I could no longer postpone deciding whether or not to have children. I had always felt that my twenties were for me to do with as I pleased, with as little responsibility as possible. Now that I was thirty, the age that represented "adulthood," and was comfortable in my work and happy with my life, I was ready to become a mother.

Like other couples committed to their work, my husband and

I planned my pregnancy to conform as much as possible to our work schedule, which for us meant the school calendar. Miraculously, I became pregnant on schedule and gave birth to a daughter three weeks after school ended. I began a year's maternity leave the following September.

———————

It is at the end of what has been a wonderfully happy and fulfilling nonworking year that I write this. Although my return to work is imminent, and I have had months to prepare Nicole and myself, I find I am ambivalent, confused, and often very depressed at the prospect of being away from my child. Instead of focusing on work, I worry about how Nicole will cope with the separation from me and from her father. I worry that not only the quantity, but the quality of my time spent with Nicole will be diminished. Will I have enough energy left after a demanding day working with other mothers' children to be patient and loving with my own child? I remember how nice it was, as a child much older than Nicole, to have my mother and grandmother constantly available to me. Will I be cheating my own child, who is so young and so dependent on adults for her care? Although I believe that Nicole will have two kind, loving, and patient caretakers (her paternal grandmother, two days a week; and home day care with a young mother for three days), I wonder who, besides me and her father, would be patient enough to let Nicole laboriously feed herself, or willing to clean up the resulting mess. I wonder if Nicole, a calm and loving child, will feel pressured by having to conform to the schedules of others, and, more painfully, whether she will feel less secure and less loved. And I am saddened for my own loss, of missing out on the many shared intimacies of our days: Nicole bringing me her favorite book to read; holding her on the rocker; being there when she looks to me with her face full of pride at a small accomplishment.

I ask myself whether or not I would be returning to work were it not for financial necessity: although my husband is now working, it looked for a time as if he would be going to law school, making me the sole support of my family for at least three years. Fears of being trapped, of not being able to leave my job even if I were convinced my daughter was unhappy, left me feeling impotent and enraged. As a feminist, I fervently believe that women should share the economic responsibility of raising a family; shouldering the entire burden was something else indeed.

Existing simultaneously with these strong feelings and concerns, however, is a desire to resume my career. I look at the children of friends who are thriving despite (or because of) good child-care arrangements and I am reassured. I reexperience how important my work is to my sense of identity and how my feelings about myself become diminished without meaningful work. I remember that, despite my love for my daughter, I do not want her to become the sole focus of all my ambitions, hopes, and dreams. Life in the Bronx left me with an overwhelming sense of wasted potential. There were many mothers whose considerable intelligence, energy, and ambition had no outlet other than cooking or being ambitious for their children. I want Nicole to have role models of women whose definition of self does not derive merely from their role as mothers.

Then there are times I simply do not want to be burdened with the tedium, the days of reading the same stories, mopping up splattered food, the circumscribed and familiar walks, and all of the plain hard work involved in a day with a young child.

I had avidly read books on pregnancy, attended Lamaze classes, and continued reading about the first year of development, so I naturally turned to these same "experts," as well as to friends, to provide insight and support for the difficult decision to return to work. While friends gladly talked of their experiences, they too often had doubts or, worse, regrets. The experts whose books were of great solace to me while I stayed home suddenly became almost uniformly disapproving now that I was to return to work. Instead of information about how to find good child care, how to help my child adjust, and what types of behavior might be expected, all I could find were reasons (few of them documented by any studies and all in complete disregard for the economic and emotional exigencies of working mothers) to stay home. That I chose to read these books says something about my willingness to shoulder all the guilt for a decision shared and supported by my husband, David. Although he is starting a new job that will demand much more of his time than his previous employment, he feels mostly pleasurable anticipation about his new work, some sadness at having less time to spend with Nicole, but no guilt.

———

My first six weeks of work have now ended. Surprisingly, Nicole and I settled quickly into a routine, and, even more surprising, there seem to be no ill effects. Occasionally Nicole will cry as I leave, but she stops before I reach the car. Both of her sitters report that she is eating well, napping on schedule, and enjoying the intermittent companionship of other children. She is very glad to see me at the end of the day, holds on furiously for the first few minutes, but then resumes her independent activities.

It is good to be working again. After four years, I still find my job interesting and satisfying. Most important, however, I am comfortable and happy with my decision to return to work. I have reaffirmed something I have always known about myself: I do not want to stay at home and be a full-time mother. I treasured my year at home and felt that it gave me time to know my child and develop my own style and rhythm as a mother. But one year was enough.

MADELINE ETTIN ISRAEL attended the High School of Music and Art, and Hunter College. She lives in a suburb of Boston, near the school system in which she is a school psychologist.

An Average Mother with an Average Job
MONICA ANN LEVIN

> *It is hard to live in the world*
> *And hard to live out of it*
> *It is hard to be one among many.*
>   — *The Dhammapada*

As the latest news feature on the successful "Career Couples" flickers on my television screen, I feel myself getting angry again. I tire of forever hearing about the exceptional. This is not what real life is about. Yes, women have the right to a career. Yes, mothers have the right to a career. But right is not always reality. I need to know about the millions of mothers who work at average jobs with average pay and have average problems. The mothers just like me.

I have a husband and two young children. I have a three-bedroom house in the suburbs, two small cars, and one large color television set. However, I do not have a hot tub and I do not jog. I do not have a maid, live-in or live-out. I do not have a mother who lives next door, down the street, or even in the same town. I do not have a maiden aunt who loves sitting for the kids. I am not a doctor, a lawyer, or a corporate executive. I am a middle-income, middle-class mother who works as a secretary.

I chose to have children, and I chose to stay home with them for nearly four years. I went back to work partly for the money, but mostly because I wanted to and needed to for my emotional well-being. As much as I love my children and enjoy them now, those initial four years at home were a living hell. I had no sense of personal fulfillment from "watching the children grow." Whatever they did, I never fooled myself into measuring my sense of achievement by their accomplishments. The reality of motherhood and child care for me was diapers and vomit. When people asked me what I did, I replied, "Nothing. I'm a mother."

Having earned money ever since I was sixteen, I couldn't stand not earning my keep. I told myself that my husband owed me for all I was doing as a mother, that I was doing a "job," but this never lessened my feelings of worthlessness. For a time I felt so inadequate that I couldn't cope with the idea of going back to work. Who would hire me? I felt dead and burned out.

Gradually things fell into place: my children were at a good developmental stage; we had moved to an area where quality day care was available; and I was offered a part-time job. I took the plunge. Once back in the work world, however, I wanted to go all the way. I wanted full-time work with full-time pay and full-time benefits. I found a full-time job but I was still dissatisfied. I felt that I should be doing something more "meaningful." I began reading the want ads again. I sent out many résumés and went on job

87

interviews for positions with titles like "Editorial Assistant," "Administrative Junior in Ad Agency," and "Junior Staff Writer." Half the jobs were secretarial with glorified titles. The other half didn't pay enough to offset the costs of day care. They had been designed for young women just out of college who have very limited expenses. So much for using my talent and education in the work world.

My quest for a career caused me to undergo a period of intense self-evaluation. I came to the conclusion that what I needed was a responsible job, not a glamorous-sounding career.

The job I settled for affords me adult company and a fair amount of intellectual stimulation from nine to five. It supplies me with anecdotes to share with my spouse and a respectable salary. It is not an upwardly mobile position; I will never be chairperson of the board. I don't need an attaché case, and I will never have an expense account. I do, however, have a measure of peace of mind.

There are realities that women with young children have to face when returning to work; they extend beyond any battle with the corporate status quo or the bilious arguments from both sides of the equal rights fence. One reality is that working mothers live with guilt — guilt from all sides.

The house is always a mess, and there is often frozen food for dinner. One of the twins has a cold and I send him or her to day care anyway, because I'll feel guilty missing a day of work for a sniffle that isn't even mine. But I feel guilty, too, because I feel guiltier about missing work than sending my child to school semi-sick. When one of my children is really sick, I stay home. Then I'm guilty because I worry about work all day. The second day their father stays home, and I sit at work feeling guilty about not being a "proper mother" and making my husband miss work (even though he makes three times what I do). And I feel guilty for feeling guilty because *Ms.* magazine says that you are supposed to fulfill yourself and not feel guilty.

The conflict between being a "responsible mother" and a "responsible employee" is never-ending. When everything is going smoothly, my mind is calm. But as soon as any extra demands are made on either front, the turmoil begins. If I am asked to work a little late, I feel lousy for refusing, but I must because my children are waiting for me. When my children ask me to participate in

88

events that occur (as they usually do) at three o'clock on Tuesday afternoon, I hate myself for saying no, but I must because I can't leave work. The pressure to be the perfect suburban mother is very strong. I *am* a suburban mother, but one who has to work. My pay check has become a necessity rather than a luxury. And I can't buy the argument that I have special privileges merely because I am a woman: I feel that I must put in a full day's work for a full day's pay, like any man.

My work situation is good. My employers and co-workers are co-operative and understanding. For the Christmas pageant, a Thanksgiving play, or a parent conference, my lunch hour is expanded. I am careful never to abuse the privilege. One advantage of having a job rather than a career is that the people I work with are also working for a living. They understand that my job is not my life. I don't lose points for caring about my family. I don't have to hide my excitement if my children do something darling. I can share my pleasure with my co-workers. On the job I work hard and do my best, but during the coffee break I do not have to pretend to read *Forbes* or the *Wall Street Journal.* I can be myself.

I feel a great sense of responsibility when it comes to my work, but my primary obligation is to my children. This is where the balancing act comes in.

Waxy yellow build-up is not dangerous to children and other living things. Cheese sandwiches and applesauce are all right for dinner. My kids wouldn't stay in bed with a little cold anyway. If they are really sick, I stay with them. I use my sick days. Heaven forbid I should ever get sick.

I have more to give to my family now that I am working. I have something to say to my husband. I do not constantly complain about being bored and useless. This makes my husband happy, which makes the children happy, which makes me happy, which makes them happy.

We share as a family more than we would if I were home. Any museum trips, lessons, or park outings have to be scheduled on weekends, which means Daddy comes along. We are doing more together as a family, and the children love it, I love it, and my husband has learned to love it.

Very often I am physically exhausted at night. Getting us all off in the morning is my responsibility. It is hectic, but somehow we manage. We have chosen to live very casually; this suits me fine, since I always hated housework. The bare necessities get done, and serious cleaning is done by teamwork on a crisis basis.

Sometimes I am very envious of the nonworking neighborhood mothers. The image of three mornings a week at the gym and a luncheon in the afternoon is often appealing, but I think that after a month of it I would shrivel up.

Sometimes I tell myself that I should have a career and claw my way to the top; that I owe it to myself and I owe it to my "sisters." Then I realize that the Superwoman syndrome is a social disease and, more important, in my innermost soul, I really have no desire to climb the ladder of corporate success. Most of us, men and women, simply have to work. Finding a pleasant, satisfying job is a great accomplishment. For me, having space in my mind and time in my life to pursue other, more personally meaningful avenues of fulfillment has been a great joy. I believe the lady-executive syndrome is a hoax for a lady with a family. I don't want to become the female version of the father in Harry Chapin's song, "Cat's in the Cradle," where my children wouldn't know me at all when they grew up.

The feminist ideology purports that fathers have to become parents, spend more time with the family, and get involved with the development of the children. I agree. But are we working mothers to abandon this parenting in favor of a three-piece suit and a private office? Not I. Many feminists would see me as having compromised. I have, but for the good of myself and my family. I will not make myself crazy for something geared to the needs of single women, and I will not be manipulated by the advertising media.

Would I like to add a maid and a hot tub to our lives? At times, of course, but that is fantasy and not at issue here. Within reality — my world as it is — I am satisfied. I hate fingerpainting, and I hate giving in to myths.

MONICA ANN LEVIN had twins when she was nearly twenty-five. She lives in Northbrook, Illinois, and works full time as an administrative secretary for a suburban board of education.

Professional and Personal Conflicts

KAREN J. SHEAFFER

"Of course, the problem centers around this mother's ambivalent feelings toward the boy," pronounced the psychiatrist in his psychological indictment of the client. My thoughts were jarred back to the preceding night when my own son woke up for the third night in a row. My husband and I no longer have enough time or energy to enjoy sex, and this particular morning we were both so tired that we snapped at each other mercilessly. My son Eben has become an intruder in our formerly happy marriage. Suddenly I have great fears for his mental health. I love him so much, but most of the time I can't stand him. "This mother's ambivalent feelings . . ." It is hard not to recognize them in myself. When Eben is four years old, will he have all the difficulties faced by the client's child? Am I being absurd to compare myself to a woman with so many problems? But many of our feelings are appallingly similar.

These doubts about my mothering creep in regularly, at times when I least expect them. I work in a mental health center with preschoolers because I enjoy it. After working half time during Eben's first year, and three-quarters time his second year, I went back full time when he turned two. I hate to admit how little I like being home with him. I look forward to picking him up after work, but on the weekends I wake up in the morning with a shudder, if it is raining and I have to spend the whole day with him. I go to work partly to get away from the fact of how difficult I find motherhood, only to hear echoes of my ambivalence once I'm there.

I still remember how uneasy I was going home from the hospital with Eben. I was frightened that I would not be able to care for him the way he needed to be cared for, and that he might even die. Perhaps I just wasn't up to the task. I pulled myself together by remembering one of my cases from the year before. The mother was quite retarded; the father was psychotic; all three children had severe health problems. Yet somehow that mother managed to keep them alive. Compared to her, my conditions for raising a child were ideal. Maybe I would make it through the first few months after all.

I quickly developed a new respect for the single, welfare mothers with whom I had worked. I had a comfortable apartment, my own wonderful mother to come and help for a week, and a husband who wanted to be with the baby and do all he could. But I still got angry, and felt abandoned and helpless, for each minute he arrived home from work later than usual. On the one night a week he went out to a meeting, I remember sitting, staring at the television with tears streaming down my face, holding our infant son and wondering how in the world any woman could manage alone all the time when I couldn't even take one evening a week. Did this mean that I would be as poor at coping with normal mothering problems as some of my clients were? Or possibly they weren't doing as badly as I had previously thought, considering their lack of supports.

In my work I meet with several day-care teachers for regular consultations. They complain about how poorly parents treat them, how parents don't understand what working in day care is like. They complain particularly about a mother who is very careless about how she dresses her child, who pins his pants together and forgets to bring changes of clothes. Apparently this woman created a big scene because they couldn't find one of her son's socks when it was time to go home. I make sympathetic noises and get them to talk more about how they are feeling, but I'm really thinking about the safety pins holding up my son's pants that day and cheering for that mother who had the nerve (or was it lack of impulse control?) to say what I've felt like saying: Why the hell do they have to lose half the stuff I send off to the day-care program? I pay enough for the care and should not have to buy new things every week as well. But having taught for several years, I remember what the day of a teacher is like, and I say nothing. After all, if they didn't care for my son, I would be the one to stay home, looking for lost socks.

When the teachers finish talking they look to me for insight into how to understand and deal with this parent. My old analysis that the mother projects her own inadequacies onto the day-care staff suddenly seems overly critical. Now that I am a mother I see it as a stale interpretation of a normal human reaction to this all-too-human state of motherhood.

―――――――

One morning I was embarrassed because I was terribly late in arriving for a meeting that I was leading for day-care directors. My two-year-old was utterly impossible that day. My husband left for work in a hurry, probably to avoid the scene he could see brewing. We could both see it: the more I pressured Eben to hurry, the more he dug in his heels; he fussed and fumed about everything. The last straw was when I got him the glass of water he had requested from the kitchen sink, and he said no, he wanted it from the bathroom. Furious, I threw the water in his face. He then fell down screaming, and I was even angrier at myself for making such a mess. I dragged him kicking and screaming out to the car, strapped him into his car seat, and ran back into the house to get my papers and lunch for work. By the time I got to work I questioned how anyone who is so incompetent that she can't even get out of the house sanely with a child could possibly be helpful to anyone else. I wanted to cry.

Incredibly, when I talked about the incident at work, no one felt that they should file a child-abuse report on me; most were quite sympathetic, while others didn't even want to be bothered hearing about such "normal" behavior from a two-year-old and his mother. It was very reassuring.

The support I get at work is helpful, but I sometimes feel that I miss out on the feedback other mothers receive because of my work. Once when I was with a group of new mothers and their young children in the park, I was feeling especially proud of my son. As one woman complimented me on Eben's friendly and co-operative behavior, another woman assured her that it was easy for me to deal with him since I was trained in working with children. . She canceled out the reassurance and support I felt from the compliment. I wanted to shout, "I need just as much support as any other mother. There is no 'training' for motherhood."

―――――――

While our son can be impossible, he can also be equally delightful. But these fun times can be anxiety provoking as well. Lately Eben and I have been developing our own little jokes and games. We pretend that we're in a cave and pull the covers over our heads. He whispers, "Now no one can find us." In the morning he gets into bed with us, carefully removes his father's hand if it's touching me, and forces his way between us. My arms encircle him and his warm, moist body is the ultimate in cuddliness. I feel flattered to have someone who is so attentive to me, so desirous of me. At work, the bubble bursts as I sit listening to a case presentation. "The issue is really this young man's unresolved feelings, precipitated by his mother's seductiveness." I wonder if my child should be in therapy. Am I ruining his future by hugging him in bed? The fact that I'm enjoying his attention should be my warning sign. Doesn't that mean that I'm really encouraging it? And isn't that what happens in cases where the marriage is no longer fulfilling? When was the last time that my husband and I talked about anything that was important to us, rather than who was going to put out the trash that week? Our life has become full of mundane necessities. Perhaps I expect my son to fill the void. I resolve to get a baby sitter for the next night so my husband and I can go out together, alone.

When things are going badly, I worry about how inadequate I am. When I'm enjoying my son, I worry about whether it's healthy for him or for my marriage. How many times have I assured other mothers that their doubts were absolutely normal, and how many times did I underestimate the pain of harboring those doubts? Becoming a mother has given me a new grasp of many of the theories I use in my work, a new compassion for many of my clients, and new insights into and anxieties about myself.

KAREN J. SHEAFFER works full time at the preschool unit of a community health and retardation center, splitting her time between a direct client case load and consulting to preschool programs in the community. She recently had a second child.

I Work Because I Have To

JANET DiVITTORIO MORGAN

Magazines are filled with articles aimed at the working woman, particularly the working mother. I am one of those working women who falls for every invitation to read an article on the "Working Mother," hoping to find one that will relate to me and to my experience. They never do.

Instead, all the articles I have found are written by or geared toward the career-oriented mother trying to cope with the responsibility of having both a child and a career. The writers, often psychologists, make every effort to assure these working mothers that there is no effect on a child who is left with a baby sitter or in day care, and that the guilt they feel is unfounded.

All I know is that I am a new mother trying to cope with the responsibility of having a nine-to-five job strictly because we need the salary. I too feel guilt because I leave my child with a sitter, even though I do it because I have to, not because I want to. I am one working mother who feels very affected by the reality of having to work full time; I resent having my motherly duties come second to the job. I feel cheated of the very time in my life for which I had longed and planned so many years.

I had always assumed that I would quit my job when I had a baby. But once that much-anticipated time arrived, our standard of living absolutely required my salary. In my heart, all I could feel was the strong desire to stay home and take care of my new baby. Because I had to go to work, I found myself blaming the job and directing all my hostility toward it.

My daily routine has taken on a dramatic change; working and having a baby are so time-consuming that my emotions are further taxed merely by the physical effort that doing both demands of me.

Since I need my job to meet our budget, hiring help in the home is out of the question. I sometimes wonder how much is expected of me. It is extremely difficult for me to wake extra early, adjust my normal routine to include feeding, dressing, and getting the baby to the sitter before I even start my day at the office. And it doesn't stop there. After finishing a hard day at work, I have the rest of the day and night to be a mother, housekeeper, cook, and laundress, not to mention wife and lover to my husband. Then it all starts again with a middle-of-the-night feeding. I am also trying somehow to make up for my day-long absence from my baby by using a sitter who is close enough to where I work to enable me to go there at lunchtime to feed the baby. The numerous new tasks in my daily routine are not causing my resentment: it's the job that has now become extra to me; it's the job that I feel is the burden.

─────────

Having to deal with a baby sitter is very painful. All I can see is another woman holding, loving, and caring for my new baby. I am actually paying her to do all the things that I wish I could be doing. I want to be able to care for my baby and am terrified at the thought of this stranger becoming important to my child (perhaps more so than I am) because of the sheer quantity of time spent with her.

Mothers are often assured that their baby instinctively senses when mothers are giving their best. I too would like to give my best to my child and worry that a bad day at the office might interfere with this.

Since this is my first child, I can only imagine what I will miss by not being with her all day. I don't want to learn my child's firsts in life from the sitter. I want those to be experiences I observe and which I share only with my husband.

It doesn't help much to appease myself with the thought that I'm working so that I can give my daughter a comfortable life or that she will save her best for me or even that the really difficult stages do not last too long. Those concepts only remind me that I am not where *I* want to be: with my daughter.

Since I do have to pacify myself with something in order to carry out this necessary but painful separation successfully, I cling to the old adage that the quality, not the quantity, of time is what counts.

JANET DiVITTORIO MORGAN has worked for eleven years in an insurance underwriting firm, formerly as a secretary and currently as a rater. The Morgans live in Sandston, Virginia.

A Working Mother

GERRI GOMPERTS

I suspect that every working mother has a recollection of the moment when it became clear to her that staying at home with her child was going to result in a prolonged stay at a mental institution. My own particular memory is one of standing in our kitchen, savagely scratching at a roll of Saran Wrap that wouldn't unroll properly, while my barely one-year-old daughter Jessie looked on. I remember the tears and my constricted throat; how mortifying to be the archetypal, neurotically depressive young mother. I was twenty-six years old, a bit "moody" as it was kindly referred to in the days of the early seventies, and overeducated. Although happily married to a man who let me breathe but also told me he loved me every day, I felt a pervasive sense of discontent which I tried tirelessly to attribute to the malaise of the times.

I had wished ardently for a daughter and she instantly became, and still is today, my heart's feast. I nursed her, rocked her, felt her become part of my nervous system in a way that no other being ever has. Yet, after the first few months, it became apparent that I had to make a decision about returning to work. I had developed a streak of manic depression that I had never before had time to explore. While Jessie napped, I brooded over my plight, my isolation, my refusal to make friends in the neighborhood, to join those groups, ever present in suburbia, designed to turn your brain into farina and your interest toward consumption. I applied to a local law school with a reputation for academic rigor and radicalism, and I was accepted.

When Jessie was eighteen months old, I left her in the care of an education major from a local college, a young woman who seemed intelligent and warm. I remember telling my husband, Victor, how conflicted I was about leaving Jessie. He smiled in his low-key way and said that he had been thinking that I was a fool to have stayed home as long as I had.

———

I did well in law school, coped with the shock of learning a new and difficult discipline, and still found time for Jessie. Contrary to

97

popular lore, I did not need to study five hours a day. I did have to accept not being first in the class; cramming murderously before an exam; saying, "I'm not prepared" when called on; and maintaining a sense of proportion. These are not easy things to learn, especially for one to whom academia had been a haven. For the first time, some sentences had to be read over and over until they made sense; exams generated an anxiety for which I was unaware I had the capacity; and I was subject to fits of guilt and depression that had never before been part of my consciousness.

Jessica was seemingly well adjusted to her baby sitter, and I came home as early as possible that first year. But I always felt of two minds: when I was home, I wanted to be studying; when I was at school, I felt a pit in my stomach at the thought of Jessie at home. I conjured up endless scenarios of child abuse, home accidents, and fatal childhood diseases visited upon my daughter for the sins of her mother.

I also began to experience the strained reactions of other women. From time to time, I would be accosted by an honest one. She would tell me straightaway, after the most cursory introduction, that anyone who would leave her child shouldn't have had one. I much preferred this to the more ambiguous and unsettling comments of the alleged admirers who would say, "I don't know how you do it." Unnerved, I would mumble about how much help I had, how my husband was so supportive, I really was home a lot, the person I left her with was . . . and on and on. Then I would go home and check Jessie for signs of incipient juvenile delinquency or leprosy.

———————————

Somewhere along the line, we decided to have a second child. We timed it with great precision so that I carried during my second year of law school and had Kate in the summer before my third year. Being pregnant in law school, so cleverly planned, increased the ranks of the seeming admirers tenfold. By now, however, I had caught on and didn't brook much of that sort of thing from the at-home mothers. After all, they lived in righteousness; they didn't need my smiles and chitchat. And pregnancy produced a palpable easing of tension in me. My appearance made me temporarily "acceptable" to the outside world, even as my intellectual commitment to a dual career grew. I felt more comfortable knowing that I did not appear to be abandoning all the traditional roles. A pregnant Germaine Greer is not threatening.

The birth of a second daughter was an unexpected treat. All signs had pointed to a boy, and I was delighted, overcome, when I heard they had all been wrong. This go-round was different. I was home only six weeks and then back at classes, svelte and confident. Katie was as good an infant as Jessie had been difficult. She was prettier, less charismatic, less verbal, more at peace in her world. I liked her but gave Jess so much that, at times, there was little left over. Jessie and I still spent much of the weekend together to make up for what I was sure she was missing all week. Now at a day-care center for her second year, she was more grown up, more of a companion, but still needy. I found her presence a constant source of wonder, but emotionally and physically draining. She was a second self. Her burgeoning sense of humor delighted me, but her moments of anguish caused me to descend into what she now calls the "pits bin."

I remember certain scenes from these years with a wrenching in my guts. Jessie at dancing school — inattentive at class, being told to follow directions, then attempting to keep up, failing, and the teacher, now in pique, her own ego flashing, making her do the steps alone, over and over. And Jessica, her head turned over her shoulder to me, mouthing, afraid to let go, "I'm so embarrassed." And only after the class broke did she run to me, her edible soft skin now white and clammy, to cry in humiliation. That look of helplessness, of fragility as she turned to me, haunts me. And then, my rage at a middle-aged, rigidly controlled woman who felt the need to be called "Miss Joan" by a bunch of six-year-olds. Did my fury rise up so fiercely because Jessica was a child being needlessly humiliated, or because I did not protect her as much as I ought to have?

We are at a cocktail party to celebrate the anticipated marriage of a medical student and a young lawyer. Many of the women are doctors or are soon to be. The rooms are decorated with African masks and sculpture. Talk is of the changing roles. I am wearing silk and silver jewelry. I stand with my back to Victor, in another group. Above the pleasant din, distinctly, I hear him. "No," he is saying, "she feels no guilt at all." A mumbled reply. Then his voice again, so unmistakably proud, "Yes, they're quite young, but she just doesn't feel guilty. Neither of us does." I move slowly through the crowd, delicately to the door. Outside, in the darkness of the bushes, I vomit, heaving and gagging. Then I walk a bit in the night shrubbery, thinking of the jagged gashes an ice pick would make around his heart.

───────────

I practice law now. I have been out there in the real world for a little over two years. I can finally say, without blushing, that I'm a lawyer (if asked directly). As John Updike says, we make our profit out of others' losses. It is not always a jolly business. I get money for people who have been hit by cars, malpracticed upon by doctors, or hurt by a product they've bought or used. I go to court, I work in the office, and, from time to time, I feel a joyful sense of accomplishment. I eke out, at best, a few laughs a day, and I cherish my sense of freedom. I stay home when one of my children is sick: I prefer it to worrying, and they prefer it to television. But I know that I do both jobs with a less-than-total commitment. It can't be helped. There are no viable alternatives. Not working is unacceptable to me. But I never read the Supermom success stories without a bitter feeling for the lies propagated. I choose to have work of my own and also to have children. It is not ideal, but it is what there is.

My mother returned to work when I was about eight years old. I knew then, as I do now, that no one in my life would love me with the depth of feeling and utter commitment to my happiness that she did. I hope my girls will feel that, despite all the logistical and often more serious inadequacies that result from the fact of having two working parents, they are loved intensely and with devotion. I hope too that they will have learned to reach for life's possibilities, so that they close off no avenues to themselves out of fear, but only out of choice.

GERRI GOMPERTS lives and practices law in New Jersey. Her husband is also a lawyer. "I am on the precipice of being thirty-three years old and cannot envision a future which would eliminate either my family or my career. However, I am sure that in my next life I shall have a greater depth of imagination."

6

*Changes
in Self-Concept*

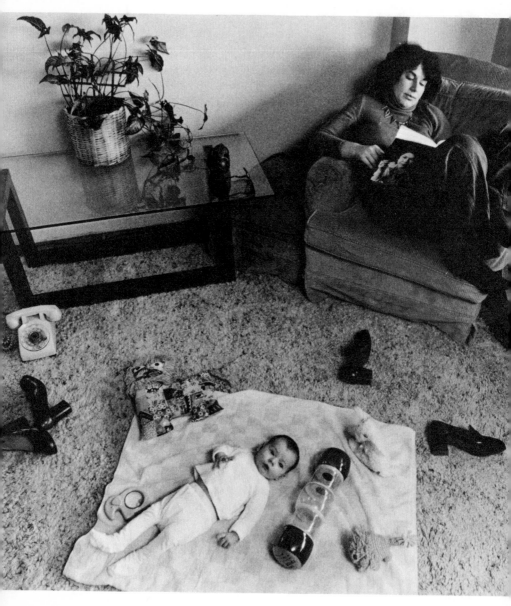

Gail LeBoff

The Emergence of a New Self-Image

RONNIE FRIEDLAND

Before the birth of my son Joshua, my self-image was that of a feminist who felt uncomfortable in the world beyond her counter-cultural circle of friends, a woman who had married late (at thirty-one) and had residual feelings of insecurity. I was a person who expected difficulties in life and feared both success and failure — one who had managed to achieve some standing in the world, but who basically had a hard time dealing with that world.

I lived in urban intellectual centers where I frequented book-stores and movie theaters. Much of my time was spent either engrossed in a book or in coffee houses engaged in leisurely discussions with friends. Although I enjoyed my lifestyle, I felt something was missing: I wanted a child.

———————

When eight-pound-one-ounce Joshua burst into my life, my world changed. No longer was my time my own. Weeks passed before I looked at a book, left my apartment, or lingered with a friend. I suddenly found myself called upon to perform whole new sorts of tasks, most of them physical or menial, yet I loved it. I've gone through a major transition, discovered new sides of myself, and the result has been the gradual emergence of a new self-image.

In contrast to the inner conflict I usually experienced in other areas of my life, I now feel integrated and at one with myself as a mother. Where previously I was often torn between incompatible urges or responses, I now feel free to rely on my instincts with my child, and I experience no contradictory impulses. I'll always remember the first time I held Joshua — and inexplicably knew exactly how to do so. In our prenatal classes we had practiced holding babies, and I had felt awkward and unsure — foreseeing the need to be taught in the hospital after he was born. But I didn't have to be taught. I just knew. I also recall how stunned a nurse was when she learned that Joshua was my first child — because I seemed so comfortable with him. This is the only area of my life where I have immediately felt competent and confident.

Those initial moments of trust in myself were reinforced on numerous occasions. Although before Joshua was born I had anticipated the need to get out on my own frequently in the first few months of motherhood, this didn't happen. I wanted to be *with* him, not away from him. This eventually led to a decision not to work for the first year, despite having thought it would be important to do so, and despite pressure to work from friends and the feminist movement, pressure I had previously exerted on others. Too much of my energy, emotions, and psyche were tied up with Joshua to leave anything over for work at that time. Occasionally during the year I missed the satisfaction provided by work, but whenever I came close to actually taking a job, I realized I was not ready to divert the time and energy from Joshua. On the whole, not working felt right and worked out well for me.

One result of not being in conflict with myself was a new sense of inner directedness. I felt much less concerned with what other people thought or felt about me, or with their advice or suggestions, whereas in the past I had to consult with friends before making major decisions. Friends have always been important to me, and they still are, but I need them less and enjoy them more.

———————

Mothering has given me the opportunity to discover new personal traits that I like and to improve on some that I don't like. Always self-critical, I had easily found a great deal in myself not to like. But part of the effect of uncritically accepting Joshua has been that I see more in *myself* that I can accept — ranging from nonintellectual virtues such as playfulness and the ability to find small things amusing to an undreamed-of ability to be patient. I surprised myself with my lack of irritation over Joshua's constant interruptions while I was trying to read the Sunday paper, and with my resigned humor when we had to race out of yet another restaurant because he couldn't sit still. Most important, discovering an ability to love uncritically and totally has been exhilarating. It's the sort of love that calls upon my whole being, bringing all of my potential to life.

It was an instinctive response to Joshua, and one I am trying to extend to my husband and to others.

Feeling comfortable and confident in motherhood has enabled me to feel more secure in my female identity. I had never felt exceptionally feminine before. Beyond an appreciation of intimacy, sensitivity to others, and a certain world view which I shared with my female friends, being a woman meant milestones to reach (get married, have a child) or dangers to avoid (don't get raped or accosted while walking down the street). Now my greatest strength springs from what I perceive as most female in me — the ability to mother — which gives my identity as a woman new depths and meaning.

This heightened sense of womanhood has strengthened my bond to that key woman in my life, my own mother. During my pregnancy and in the early months of motherhood my ties to my mother preoccupied me. I spent hours analyzing and discovering our similarities, imagining her experience as a mother and my experience as her child. Although this preoccupation has passed and our differences in style and personality have once again become more central, my new and deepened appreciation of what it means to be a mother has created a bond which will, I believe, remain.

This bond extends beyond my mother to all other mothers and pregnant women. It is rooted in the universal aspects of every mother's experiences and concerns. And this sense of connection with other mothers — both young and old — is a wonderful addition to my life. How strange for a person like me, who always considered herself an outsider, suddenly to feel on the inside, in the mainstream, and sharing what is most important in my life with what is important to most other women. Before Joshua was born I only felt comfortable with an extremely narrow range of people who had similar values, ideals, and outlooks, but motherhood has enabled me to connect with a whole new spectrum of people — those who have families. My interests and priorities have also changed. Whereas my favorite pastime was watching foreign films, now I also enjoy sitting on the front stoop, talking to other mothers while our kids chase each other down the block. Whereas before my main interest in a neighborhood was its access to restaurants, movie theaters, and shops, now I am concerned also with schools, parks, and playgrounds.

My central goal, the one thing that never altered despite the many changes and radical stages I went through in the sixties, was to have a child. Having had one, I can now relax and enjoy life, feeling less pressured by time. Until I had Joshua at thirty-three, I had perceived time as an enemy, running out, and I felt pressured to conceive before I turned thirty-five. Now time is less of a threat, and birthdays are no longer so depressing. I feel fulfilled, having satisfied my deepest yearnings as a woman and as a human being.

Now that I feel better about my personal life, I can step back and reevaluate my professional goals. I feel freer to reject an unsatisfactory job teaching English composition at a local college and finally to leave college teaching altogether to seek a career more suited to my present needs and interests. Before Joshua, it was too difficult to admit I was in the wrong field, because too much of my self-esteem was tied up with my career, and it was too threatening to be overly successful in my career because it might prove that I was a "career" person instead of a "woman." Now, however, I feel satisfied enough in motherhood to look more closely at my career needs and dissatisfactions, and to make changes.

A precious effect of having had a child is that I now perceive myself as a relative success in life, a perception that alters my whole sense of self and affects every moment of my life, my reflections, and my interactions with the world. My previous sense of being unfulfilled as a woman was a burden that interfered with my relationships with new people and my work. Now that I am free of it, my interactions with other people are more positive and less taxing. Despite my feminist belief that every woman need not have a child to be complete and to feel fulfilled, in my own case having one was necessary and enriched my life immeasurably.

RONNIE FRIEDLAND and her husband happily shared parenting for the first year of her two-year-old son's life. They then returned to their career pursuits — he teaching philosophy, and she working on this book. "I discovered that despite interruptions I work best when a sitter cares for Joshua in our home: Hearing his frequent peals of laughter relieves me of any anxieties about him."

Lazarus as Mother: Returning from Depression

NAOMI KAPLAN

> *"I am Lazarus, come from the dead.*
> *Come back to tell you all, I shall tell you all."*
> — T. S. Eliot

I have traced the inception of the postpartum depression I experienced for the first two years of my son's life to the moment I first learned of my pregnancy — from an anonymous voice over the phone. I had dreaded making that call. Married less than two years, my husband and I had frequently discussed starting a family, but we both felt that we wanted a bit more time to develop our own relationship and to establish ourselves more securely in our professions. Upon hearing the confirmation of my pregnancy, my first thought was, What am I going to do about my special education students? My second thought was, What will I do if *my* child turns out to be a "problem child" like those students?

Contributing to my anxiety was the sense that I was soon going to turn thirty and that my "time was running out" to glut myself with the adventures, experiences, and accomplishments I had fantasized about since I was an adolescent. I especially feared losing my carefree lifestyle. No longer would my husband and I be able to go hiking or skiing for a weekend, or see a double feature at the spur of the moment; for years we would be denied much of our treasured private time together.

I felt that the qualities my husband enjoyed most about me — spontaneity, gregariousness, and spirit — would all be lost for the next two decades, during which I would be transformed into an uninteresting drudge. I remembered my shock when, as an adolescent, I found an old photo of my mother — beautiful and glamorous as a movie star — dancing with my handsome father, before they were married. I couldn't believe that this was the frazzled, overweight person who was my mother. I longed to emulate that exciting woman in the photo — not the tired housewife wiping noses. My pregnancy made me think that the latter was my inevitable destiny.

Although I had led an interesting, eventful life filled with travel and a variety of jobs and relationships, I felt I had not yet achieved very much. How would I now be able to write the Great American Novel or at least become a master teacher — with a baby consuming my time and energy? Pregnancy became a time of self-appraisal, and I discovered that I didn't add up to much.

Despite these sentiments, I also had positive feelings about my pregnancy. When I felt the baby move and kick, I was thrilled; I dreamed of holding him in my arms and nursing him. I had always liked children, and I looked forward to exploring the world and to sharing the things I loved — poetry, music, movies, books — with my own child.

As the pregnancy progressed, I became more and more confused by the ambivalence of my emotions. My feelings were a mass of contradictions. As my due date approached and my anxiety mounted, I began seeing my therapist three times a week instead of one; I withdrew from shopping trips that involved purchasing any baby clothes or equipment; I talked endlessly on the phone with women about the value of having children; and I read repeatedly and obsessively the statistics on birth defects and abnormalities. My awareness of my own body became distorted: at times I thought the baby was too small; the next day I would be convinced that I was expecting twins.

And all the while, the question of what to do about my job plagued me. Finally I decided to return to work full time three weeks after the baby was born. My husband, who was self-employed, agreed to stay home and be the primary care giver. The ease with which this problem was resolved dazzled and exhilarated me. I harbored the illusion that my life would change very little after all, and that I would not be cut off from the world I loved. Even before the baby was born, I felt guilty over my eagerness to be away from home, but I pushed these feelings into the recesses of my awareness. There the guilt remained, only to surface later to the point where it debilitated me.

Our baby emerged healthy and perfectly formed, after a quick, easy delivery. During a restful and comforting hospital stay, I was continually assured that all was fine and that I was handling everything beautifully. But what was there to handle? I merely fed the baby and held him. The nurses changed him, bathed him, and put him to bed. They took him back to the nursery when I was tired or had company. Motherhood, apparently, was simple.

I came home to find my mother more than willing to assume the nurses' duties. But ten days later she departed to her own home hundreds of miles away, and I was on my own. And afraid.

From that point on, things began to go wrong. I developed mastitis three times, and for a month was on heavy dosages of antibiotics which made me tired and nauseated. It seemed that I could never get enough sleep, get caught up with the laundry, or cook a complete meal. And I was so unsure of how to take care of a baby that I thought he should be held and "stimulated" during all his waking moments in order for him to develop normally. My husband was extremely helpful and supportive during this period, but that in itself became a mixed blessing: he gladly changed and bathed the baby, brought him to me for the two-in-the-morning feedings, amused him, cooked, cleaned, and even did the laundry. He did all these tasks so effortlessly and cheerfully that I began to feel incompetent and inadequate as well as guilty that I was constantly (and eagerly) relinquishing my role to him.

It made me increasingly anxious that what seemed so simple to my husband was becoming very difficult for me. I did not know how to interpret the baby's cries; I didn't know how often to change him, and I was always afraid of either underfeeding or overfeeding him.

Our pediatrician laughed off my unending barrage of questions and attributed my mounting anxiety to nothing more than "new-mother nervousness." I had virtually no friends with children, and I was lonely and isolated from my friends at work. As I grew more estranged from my former life, I became more frightened and depressed by my inability to handle my new life.

I had to postpone returning to work because of the bouts of mastitis. When I did return several weeks later, I was on antidepressant medication, and preoccupied with unfulfilled duties at home. I could not function effectively at my job, and I was asked to leave. This was a devastating blow to me, for my job was my only remaining tie to the outside world. With that gone too, my depression intensified.

Since I was at home full time, my husband returned to work. I was alone all day, housebound by a snowy, cold winter. Friends dropped by occasionally, but I could not hold a conversation without alluding to my sadness. I was angry at myself for boring them, yet I wanted their help. Eventually they stopped coming.

My husband began to stay home more frequently; by the time the baby was about two months old, he was at home constantly. I was terrified to stay alone with the baby even if my husband left the room for only a few minutes. I kept my husband up for hours each night trying to talk out and analyze my burgeoning feelings of confinement, ineptitude, and loss. I kept explaining to him, night after night, that I was completely panicked about being a mother, and that to me being a person and being a mother were incompatible. It seemed as though all my connections to my former self were totally severed and I was foundering helplessly in a new self that was not me; indeed this self was so different that it was as if I were living someone else's life, or that I was having a distorted nightmare from which I could not escape. And I couldn't wake up and find that it was over — because I *was* awake. There was no way out except one: I began to talk of suicide. My husband listened and tried to be supportive, reassuring me that my sadness would pass. But he was unable to grasp the reality that I could not be "pep-talked" out of my depression.

Even my psychiatrist could not handle this constant state of crisis. Instead, she focused on my early childhood, rattling on about anal fixations. But it was not the past that tormented me — it was the present.

During this period I needed to be constantly on the go, moving about, visiting people, driving or walking aimlessly, busying myself with endless activities to stave off my feelings of despair. I was desperately trying to conjure up my former blithe, carefree self again, but I just could not retrieve it.

One day as we drove to visit friends, I began speeding wildly. My husband was holding the baby and screaming for me to stop. The incident terrified both of us. We realized that although I did not actually want to destroy myself and my family, I could no longer keep up the pretense of normal functioning and was trying to express my desperation.

When we reached our friends' home, I nursed the baby, tears rolling down my cheeks. I asked my friend how she managed and how she could have given up a job she loved. She responded that her daughter was the "joy of her life" and that she found her new life "difficult but rewarding." I could not really understand and she could not really explain. It was just a "feeling," she said. She was right. It *was* a feeling. You either had it or you didn't, and it seemed to me that I, for the most part, didn't.

After I finished nursing the baby, I bolted out the door. I ran around the block several times by myself, "enjoying" a few minutes of solitude and freedom. My husband sat with our friends and broke down and cried, realizing at last that his fantasy of a happy family life was not to be and that I needed to be hospitalized.

But we continued the pretense of being a family for a few more weeks, until the pressure became unbearable for me. In my husband's presence, I tried to overdose. A part of me wanted to die; another part wanted to be rescued. But both parts wanted the suffering to end. I lay on the floor screaming that I could not go on and that I wanted to die. My psychiatrist, who had merely been upping my dosage of antidepressants and denying any need for hospitalization, finally secured a room for me in a psychiatric ward.

Being hospitalized was a great relief, probably subconsciously corresponding to my pleasant experience in the maternity ward: the baby stayed in another part of the hospital during the day with my mother-in-law and was brought in to me for his feedings. But being in that ward, with an assortment of people with whom I had no connection, shared feelings, or experiences, was also somewhat alienating. I also had difficulties relating to my new psychiatrist, a young man who I felt could not understand my problems with adjusting to motherhood since he was not a mother.

Problems began to arise with my mother-in-law, who would sit in my room while I nursed the baby, telling me how well *she* had been able to manage five children and a full-time career, and how simple this all could be for me. She neglected, however, to acknowledge the fact that she had had servants and a governess — a vital support system which I lacked. She also interfered with my precious time alone with the baby, which I had begun to look forward to since the twenty-four-hour-a-day pressure of caring for him had been relieved. She undermined my already low confidence in myself and in my ability to be a good mother. Once, as I nervously began to feed the baby some cereal, he started coughing. "He's choking," she shouted and snatched him from me. This image has never faded from my mind. It epitomized the hypocrisy that I felt surrounded me: everyone said I could be a good mother, but no one gave any evidence of believing it.

On the whole I improved while in the hospital — I felt less depressed and anxious and more able to cope. I was released six weeks later. But when I returned to our hot, dingy apartment and to the same situation I had left, I also reverted to my former psychic state. I was rehospitalized two months later. My mother, who continued to be very supportive throughout this ordeal, then returned to take care of the baby while I was hospitalized.

This was the pattern that was to be repeated over the next eighteen months: hospital after hospital, shrink after shrink, medication after medication. The process was cyclical: I would come home and attempt to manage my life, only to grow more depressed each day and more hopeless about the possibility of resuming my career. Then more anxiety. More guilt. Helplessness. Rehospitalization.

When the baby was about a year old, he was moved to my in-laws' home while my husband continued to live with me. Although the seeming source of pressure (the baby) had been removed, the essential feelings of loss, inadequacy, and guilt persevered. Nearly a year passed in this fashion until my husband could stand the separation from our son no longer. So he separated from me.

I became suicidal again and needed to be rehospitalized. My husband found that no private hospitals were willing to admit me unless they had locked wards. These apparently were full, so he decided that I should go to a state hospital. My parents immediately flew up to see what else could be done. They and my extended family mobilized their efforts to get me into a private hospital. My husband and his family offered very little assistance in this, and their lack of support depressed me further.

After finally being admitted to a private hospital, I was given various forms of therapy and medication, but nothing seemed to help. My parents and I met with my psychiatrist to determine how my treatment should proceed. I walked around the room, refusing to sit down, wringing my hands and crying. It was obvious to all of us how desperate I was. It was clear that nothing had worked thus far. In my career as a mental patient, I had run the gamut of diagnoses: everything from psychosis to hormone imbalance. No matter what the diagnosis or treatment, however, I had remained in essentially the same condition for nearly two years.

My psychiatrist, who had conferred with other doctors who had treated me, recommended shock treatments as the most effective way of quickly relieving the despair and distress I was experiencing. He explained the pros and cons, and although distraught, I was rational enough to realize that while shock treatments had been subject to a bad press, they were, for me, the last resort. I agreed to undergo them. It was the first decision I had made on my own since the onset of my depression — my first decision without my husband, his family, or psychiatrists. I was rather proud of myself for taking this seemingly small step.

As soon as I began receiving the shock treatments, I improved dramatically. I wanted to see the baby. I began to interact with the staff and patients (instead of pacing around and wringing my hands). I was more receptive to psychotherapy. The depression began to lift.

I was released from the hospital two months later, feeling relaxed and self-confident enough to begin the process of taking care of my family at last. The irony, of course, was that there was no family to care for: my husband had moved into his parents' home with our child. Fortunately, my parents decided to stay with me for a few months. Their presence and continued emotional support were major factors in promoting my recovery. Their faith in my ability to mother my son, and their availability for listening, talking, and just "being there," gave me much of the strength and self-assurance I needed to counteract the losses I had suffered. I had few friends by this point, and my husband's family had regressed from coldness toward me to outright rejection. If my parents had not been there, offering constant reassurance, I am not sure that the precarious balance of my mental health would have been maintained.

I began visiting my son once a week, then two and three times weekly. He was another reason that my recovery stabilized. Relating to an infant had been arduous and boring, but interacting with an imaginative, verbal two-year-old was exciting and fascinating. Also, he was able to relate and respond to *me,* which made me feel that at last I must be doing *something* right as a mother.

I began to feel well enough to work again, and I found a part-time teaching job. Knowing that I could function in the working world was another boost to my battered ego. I was now able to cope on a part-time basis with two essential parts of my life — working and mothering.

My husband and I slowly began to reestablish our relationship. We started "dating" and getting to know each other again, a necessary step, since we both had been transformed by the experiences we had undergone in the last two years. There were distances between us and fears on both our parts: he was afraid that I might have another relapse; and I was afraid that he would never completely believe that I had recovered. At times I was not sure if I could trust him to care for me adequately: would he support my need to be out of the house for both work and amusement or would he interpret this as a rejection of motherhood? Would he suspect every sign of discontent as a harbinger of depression? And if I did get depressed again, would he put me in a state hospital? These questions troubled me. Nonetheless, after a year's separation, he moved back to our house with our son.

───────────

Now that we are together again, we are each trying to work out a satisfying personal and family life. At times we find this balance, and at times we feel a certain alienation from each other caused by those two years of mental illness and one year of separation. But our sense of commitment to each other and to being a family is strong — and a great bond between us.

Being a mother is still sometimes a strain, but there are enough compensations to reward and satisfy me. My feelings about motherhood are more balanced. Although I still feel ambivalent and overwhelmed occasionally, these sensations are fleeting. This is due, I feel, to enjoying the time my son and I spend together, seeing that I am contributing to the development of a happy, charming child, and realizing that motherhood has, in fact, not prevented me from having time and space for myself. I am continuing to teach part time, working on a master's degree, and spending time with my husband and my friends. An equilibrium now exists that allows me to be both a mother and a separate individual.

Now that more of my friends are also mothers, I realize that they too are occasionally overwhelmed and frustrated. This has dispelled much of the self-recrimination, isolation, and anxiety that plunged me into such a state of despair when my son was an infant. I accept the fact that for me being a mother may never be like the idealized world of a Mary Cassatt painting, but instead more like an unfinished expressionist canvas. It may never be idyllic, but no longer does it need to be. I have found my own style.

NAOMI KAPLAN is a pseudonym.

Merging Versus Submerging Self with Motherhood

CATHY SLOAT SHAW

Shortly after the birth of my daughter, I became aware of the lack of harmony between my operational outside self and my inner being. The mother self was the functioning body, and it was capable, competent, relaxed, and totally devoted to the care of Emily. It read book after book on child care and responded instantly to her slightest whimper. The other self was fragmented, confused, and flitted around just beyond my grasp.

I was so aware of the new life I had brought into the world that I lost contact with my own needs. I felt chagrin when at my six-week postpartum checkup I had still not healed, and despair when I had not recovered three months later.

It seemed impossible simply to rest and repair. I was unable to take charge of my body or to organize my life. Not only was it difficult to concentrate on my physical needs, but it was hard to feed my intellectual and emotional selves as well.

────────────

Strangers, neighbors, acquaintances, and relatives relegated me to caretaker of the baby and marveled at her perfection. After a perfunctory look at my hollow-eyed and still-plump body bulging out from too-small clothes, they would ask sweetly if she looked just like her father, implying that I was no more than a vessel for her birth. Pictures would be pulled from family albums to prove the fact that undeniably she was the precise replication of this relative or that. Even while categorizing me, they denied me the pleasure of creation.

Copious questions were asked about the details of her everyday existence, and when that was exhausted, the questioner would depart or turn away to seek more interesting discussion.

The same pattern repeated itself at parties or even in meeting old friends. Somehow I was no longer perceived as the same person, and my sphere of interest was assumed to go no further than my daughter's world. Often, after questioners exhausted their repertory of concerns about Emily, they would turn to my future, asking when we planned to have the next child.

I realized that these questions were voiced with interest, and often with love, but I felt frustrated by my new image as mother, restricted to a tightly defined world. The parameters were not set by me but by others, and I felt thrust into a corner. It was a space bound by limiting assumptions: Mothers must be devoted solely to their children; they can no longer function as nonmothers in the outside world.

Initially I fought this segregation by taking the baby everywhere. With her in her front pouch, snuggled up against my warmth, we traveled once again as one. The effort to get out and resume life's functions, however, was grueling. My baby was a large one (over ten pounds at two weeks), and being only five-foot-two, I found my body aching under the strain of carrying baby and the large bag of paraphernalia that always accompanied us.

Our forays into the adult world were viewed with lip-service admiration but quick disapproval if Emily behaved in nonadult ways. I keenly felt the limits put upon us by the exclusionary tactics of the adult world. For example, toilet facilities were few and far between, and those available never provided changing areas. Crossing the street with Emily on my hip and her urine trickling down my legs, a warm wetness fouling my dress, further increased my sense of distance from the downtown nonparent bustle surrounding me and my infant.

When the snows came, the strain of intruding on the adult world became greater, and I began to seek out other new mothers for companionship.

I quickly became immersed in a community of mothers which was almost startling in its warmth and acceptance of the realities of babies. Days were planned around sleeping and feeding needs. Meeting in informal groups, the babies lolled on the floor together, and mothers relaxed around them, sharing experiences of mothering with one another.

As my network of mother friends grew, I was drawn into more and more activities. My days seemed almost frantically filled. I was constantly going places with other mothers or talking on the phone, making arrangements to go. In the midst of this whirlwind of activity, I suddenly realized I was trapped in the deadening middle, the quiet center, as everyone swirled around me.

I noticed I lacked interest in the very activities that consumed my day. Meeting with mother after mother had a wearying sameness to it. I didn't care enough about each function of my daughter to dwell on it in depth. I wanted her well fed, diapered, and warmly clad, but I couldn't discuss details of it.

I noticed that I daydreamed at friends' houses and felt floaty and removed from my body. While I was seeking out people to avoid isolation, ironically I was feeling more alone than ever.

Sometimes I itched with a strange restlessness bubbling up inside; other times I turned melancholy and tears would spring to my eyes for no apparent reason. I felt violently, aggressively moody, but most of all I felt out of touch with myself and what it was I was seeking.

I was so disjointed that I had difficulty expressing myself — it was as if I were on a drugged high, and in a sense I was. Fatigue was constantly draining me. The three months of infections following my daughter's birth were finally gone, but months of tiredness, coupled with constant awakenings throughout the night, dragged on. I was tired and fragmented and no longer capable of driving myself by sheer force of will.

I decided that my bodily needs would assume first priority and that I would worry about fragmented mental selves later. Every afternoon I lay down and shared a nap with my daughter. I disentangled myself from baby-sitting cooperatives and play-group activities. As I started feeling physically healthier, I noticed a new alertness returning. I became more rational, and more capable of verbalizing my swirling emotions.

The uneasy feeling that I no longer mattered as a person, but only as a mother, had been plaguing me for months. I felt that I had been forced to take a quantum leap away from self-concerns and needs, and just self-being. A new person had come into being whose presence so dominated me that I found it difficult to remember who I had been or what I had done before her life had formed.

Babies are all ego, and their demands are immediate and total. Babies are also taxing bosses who dictate the hours of work, and the conditions. The most difficult adjustment I had to make was getting used to the total absence of personal time, the absence of quiet space.

I was doubly shocked because my difficulties brought to the forefront two mythical preconceptions that I had carried along with my pregnancy. First, I had thought that caring for a baby was a relatively easy job which would give me ample time to do everything I had never had a chance to do while working full time. I would finally be able to go back to school in a doctoral program, learn to draw, improve my photography, work on handmade quilts, grow and can my own produce, work part time, and of course care lovingly for my baby. Second, I felt that if I did nothing but stay home with Emily, I would stagnate and lose all vitality. Both ideas propelled me, and neither was realistic.

The more time Emily consumed, the more I flagellated myself over what I was not doing. It seemed to give me an almost perverse pleasure to find something else that I felt was a failure on my part, from not fertilizing the tomatoes by a certain date to being too tired to read books.

I was not satisfied with staying with mother friends all day, and yet I found it difficult to accomplish any of my goals with Emily at my side. I was not aware of what was troubling me, only that I felt deep disappointment in myself and in my abilities.

With the help of a loving husband, mother, and friends, I was able to step back from two disparate selves and review my life. I realized how I had absorbed an image of a Superwoman in a largely unconscious manner. I kept measuring myself against an ideal Supermom who cared beautifully for six children, ran her own business, and prepared lavish picnics on weekends. Surely with one small girl, I should be able to do at least as well. I also began to realize that my preconceptions of babies had been wildly off target. I had imagined them as children who were easily soothed, napped on schedule for large chunks of the day, and listened to records and played with mobiles when awake. The reality was quite the opposite: my daughter wanted to be in my arms constantly, and her needs consumed my day.

Of my two selves, I found that the Cathy self was the lost, troubled one. It made list after list of things to do or to accomplish, all of which provided tangible rewards for the doer. Concrete rewards are what I had been used to. Having worked simultaneously during most of my extensive education, my accomplishments had always been marked by completing a paper or a work day, with grades and pay checks thrown in to sweeten the reward.

Life as a mommy was incredibly different. Even with a husband who shouldered household responsibilities, as mine did, child/housework stretched on. The limits of mothering have no bounds: babies wake often during the night, and care is determined by their needs, not yours. I remember one time when the three of us had stomach flu. The only thing that soothed Emily was rocking, which nauseated me further. We rocked from four in the morning until dawn, with occasional screaming breaks, since I had to put her down every time I ran to the bathroom to vomit. There was no one I could call to say I wouldn't be at work/school today because I had the flu. The job is all-encompassing: it trails behind you even when you are sick or the baby sitter takes over.

I approached mothering in the same spirit with which I had approached all challenges in the past: demand a lot of yourself, and everything will get accomplished with hard work and energy. What I failed to understand was that the birth of my daughter demanded a lot more from me than that. Being a mother changes the previous realities. My major problem was failing to see motherhood as a difference in essence, not just in kind. I changed with the birth of my daughter, and that evolution continued after her arrival. Having a baby means merging part of yourself with another. After the initial union of sperm and seed, I believed that the melding of flesh was over; I had expected to revert back to original form after Emily's birth, but my very needs and self had altered.

I wanted to continue to grow as a person, but I also needed to grow as a mother. I finally began to alter the structure of my days, to make the most of the time available. I continued to spend lots of time with other mothers, but I began to form friendships on the basis of mutual interests beyond children and proximity. I stopped doing cleaning during Emily's naps, and used that time to do something I really wanted to accomplish. As for my professional goals, I switched the job I had started right after Emily's birth, from six hours a week interviewing new mothers after childbirth to twelve hours a week creating a library for a state agency.

Before Emily's first birthday, I felt my two selves slide back into one. There was a harmony in my body that had not been there for some time. I no longer moved at the pace I once did before her appearance, nor did I berate myself for unaccomplished tasks. Rather, I let the days assume their own flow and found them far more rewarding.

The day after her daughter's birth, CATHY SLOAT SHAW accepted a job interviewing women about their pregnancy experiences for a hospital study. She eventually overdosed on mother experiences and when Emily was one, she began and continues to work part-time as a library consultant for the Massachusetts Commission for the Blind.

Redefining Relationships: Husband

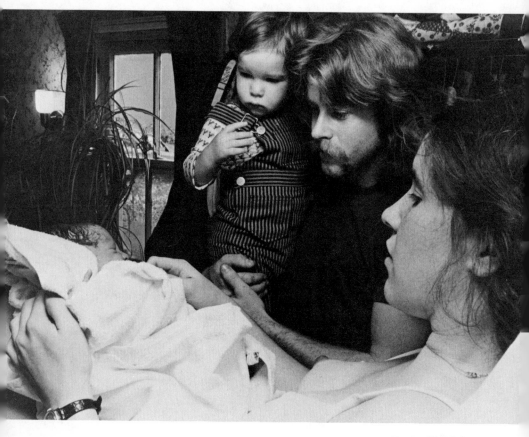

Peggy McMahon

Primal Bond Versus Marriage Bond

CAROL KORT

For the first several weeks after my daughter was born, I was over-weight, overtired, and overburdened. I had little feeling for my husband and certainly no time for my relationship with him. I had been told by the dozen books sitting on the shelf near the crib that this was perfectly normal. But as those initial weeks turned to months, and then more months, I became concerned. Where was my sexuality? Where was my husband?

The books all said that at six weeks post-birth, the mother can resume "normal sexual relations." The last thing in the world I felt was sexy. Still, I made the obligatory appointment with my gyne-cologist to have my diaphragm refitted. While she discussed the size of my cervix with me, my mind wandered to how Eleza was faring with a new baby sitter. I tried to think about sensuality and lust, but in fact my thoughts kept returning to getting home in time for the next nursing, ordering a washing machine, and buying a bottle of liquid Tylenol. I was totally out of touch with my physical desires, except to nurse, and only in touch with what was expected of me in my new role as a mother.

For weeks I had been unable to lend support or to give feedback to Michael as to how he was doing as a new father. I was not there to comfort him in his exhaustion or to allay his fears about provid-ing for our child. I felt guilty and frightened that I was having so little to do with my husband, but my physical and physiological bonds were with my daughter, and no other.

I had only enough energy to concentrate on myself and on getting through the days that had no names, and the nights that had no sleep. Sometimes I would be aware that Michael was next to me in our bed, but all I could experience was jealousy that he could sleep through Eleza's wails and that I could not; or that my breasts were painfully filling from an overdue feeding while his body was strong and lean and normal. He would be running and shopping and doing, while I sat home on a ridiculous rubber tube and rocked our daughter to sleep, trying to ignore the episiotomy that was taking about eight weeks to heal, and the hemorrhoids that plagued my every step. Having experienced a glorious pregnancy and easy delivery, it was a come-down to be at the mercy of such nonspiritual, mundane protuberances.

Nothing I had read had prepared me for the physical exhaustion and discomfort and how they would drain and deplete me of my normal drives. I could not resume "normal relations" of any kind, whether they were sexual or connected with work, friends, or family. When the plaintive, hungry cries of my infant filled the corridors of our home in the dead of night, I had but one desire — to sleep.

―――――――――

There were many changes in my relationship with my husband during those early, post-delivery months. I am the type of person who usually faces everyday difficulties calmly and coolly. I am independent in spirit and able to cope with most things tossed my way without having to discuss matters with friends, or with Michael. Prior to Eleza's birth, when Michael and I argued, I would fantasize leaving him. Oh yes, it would be sad and horrible; after all, we have been good friends and lovers for over a decade. But in that fantasy I felt perfectly capable of getting into a car and zooming away to find someone, or something, else.

Immediately after our child was born, however, I experienced a new dependence. Not only could I not just pick up and go as far as the local grocery, but during those early months I could not imagine getting through a single day or night without his help. Eleza vitally needed us both, and we needed each other to help with her. I also needed him to take care of me. During those first months, then, it was not my feelings of love or desire for Michael, but my feelings of need that bound us together.

Because Eleza was colicky for the first two months of her life, I was often weak and despondent from her constant screaming. I remember one day, when she was recovering from an attack of colic, and I was desperately hugging her tense little red body, Michael came over and held me in his arms. That was all, but it was poignant merely to be nurtured — to have someone comforting me, and not the baby. Even more than the sleep I craved, the silence I longed for, or the advice I sought, I needed that loving hug from my husband.

But mostly during that early period, the bonding process with Eleza precluded strong or passionate feelings for anyone else, including Michael. I was madly in love, quite literally, with my new daughter. I would actually overlook Michael, although he was physically right there; I could not have cared less. I would see him as if he were a spirit moving around in the same dwelling, but not really there as a person. My daughter and I had a three-dimensional reality: everyone else had become two-dimensional and unreal for me.

I was too exhausted to even wonder how Michael was feeling living with a zombie. He was consistently helpful and cheerful, and he was a good father; but we never talked about how we felt as husband and wife during that period.

While my relationship with my husband suffered, my feelings for my mother grew. When Eleza was one week old, and my mother was visiting us to help with the baby, I felt closer to her than I ever have before or since.

While my mother was with us, Eleza came down with a case of thrush. It may sound like a Chinese bird, but in fact it is a nasty yeast infection of the mouth. Although thrush is common and easily treated, upon being presented with the news that my one-week-old infant had "something," I burst out crying. I was frightened: the protector who already could not protect. And it was the comfort of my mother, not my husband, that I sought. I was also the daughter who was tired and needed reassurance that everything would be all right. My mother told me to take a hot bath and relax, and that Eleza would be fine. It may not have been the most scientific remedy in the world, but at the time it was exactly what I needed: to be told what to do; to be a daughter instead of a mother for a few moments; and to have my mother do some mothering.

Michael was not part of this scenario. He was not part of the generational link of mother to daughter to her own daughter. He was the outsider, and I perceived him that way.

Those difficult, early months after the birth of our child, interminable as they seemed at the time, passed. Eleza became less demanding and much happier. Her colic diminished, her sleeping habits improved, and she was learning to channel her energy into play and communication. Slowly I began to work other relationships back into my life. And slowly, after that period of barely "seeing" Michael, I began to see and admire him in his new role. He gave our daughter things that I could not. He was loving and tender with her, but he also played rougher. He was devoted and gentle, but he would discipline her in ways that I never could. I learned to respect him as a father, as I had respected him as my partner. I never felt or feel jealous that Eleza might prefer him for a certain game, or time of day; we each take active but different roles in what we give to and get from our child.

And there was something else very crucial that brought us together again: we shared a bond to someone that no one else had; there was a certain area in our lives that was mutually and exclusively ours. Once Eleza was doing more than merely screaming or sleeping, I wanted to talk endlessly about our adorable and clever little petunia blossom. Who else but Michael was as interested in her as I? Who else but my husband could appreciate the subtle changes that go unobserved by all others? I was newly connected to Michael, through Eleza, in a powerful way. And this family-self humbled me and brought me a deeper awareness of my purpose on earth.

The fact that Michael and I shared this rich and remarkable experience has strengthened us as individuals and as a couple. Having a child ultimately brought us closer together, after an initial period of several months during which we were very far apart. I do not regret those first months of letting go of my relationship with Michael. Our child took all we had to give, and she had a birthright to that time and space. Fortunately our relationship was strong and solid enough to survive a period of total neglect. For us, it was only a temporary separation. But at the time I only knew that I felt nothing for him, and it was therefore disconcerting.

Michael and I had waited almost ten years to have a child; I was twenty-three when I married. I never dreamed that I would be an "older" mother; in fact, for many years I never thought that I would be a mother at all. But being older has enabled us to be ready for parenthood, and I believe we are better parents because of it. If we had been young parents, I don't know if our relationship could have weathered the storm of the postpartum months. We are more able to accept and to resolve differences and crises at this time in our lives.

My return to Michael was a return to my needs. Just as I had attended my seedling and nourished her, so now I am attending seeds of my own — my professional life, my interests, and my relationship with my husband. Whereas all voices were pushed aside to hear Eleza's voice in the night, or her laughter at play, I now hear voices from the outer world. I am a mother; but I am again a wife, friend, working woman, lover, writer, and dreamer: in short, a full person. My mad crush on Eleza has turned into a restrained but powerful love affair that allows me to give to others.

Michael and I are able to share moments that belong to the two of us, not to the three of us. I have taken Eleza into my soul, but I have again made room for others, and for myself.

As our child grows into a beautiful, sometimes delightful toddler, I too have grown and have once again reclaimed my partner in marriage. I will never, however, forget those first sleepless months when I felt so alone, except for my throbbing, primal ties with my daughter. Michael was not a part of those memories, neither the good nor the bad ones.

We have not attempted to step backward to recapture our prechild relationship. That would be impossible. But we have, I believe, come out with a synthesis that has brought a new dimension to the relationship.

Becoming a mother changed every fiber, every feeling, and every relationship for me. I am constantly in the process of evaluating, recognizing, and repudiating the effects of the upheaval of motherhood. It is not a time to deal alone with the conflicts and problems; it is not a time to exist in a vacuum. I had to withdraw from Michael; and I had to return again to my closest friend.

I used to be amazed that I could grow a child. Now I am amazed that she is growing beyond me, and that I am growing beyond her.

"I am always small but shrink when challenged, melting away vertebrae, retracting my neck like an upturned tortoise / I would make a dreadful mother, I tell my mother / She says no, knowing not how small I am." So began a poem *CAROL KORT* wrote ten years ago. Today, *"I meet more challenges and see that I am not a dreadful mother: I am a normal one. I have my good days; I have my bad days."*

The Mother-Son-Husband Triangle

ALICE JOHNSON

I knew that the pattern of our lives would alter with the birth of our son. How could it not? He was a new person, with new requirements, making for new routines. I was ready for those disruptions; however, I did not expect my relationship with my husband to change. My husband was not prepared for any readjustments, although he said, and thought, that he was. As the days passed and our lives did become different, I could see resentment growing between us, driving us apart. He resented David, and I resented him for feeling that way.

When David was born, Bob was proud of him. At least I think he was. It is very hard for him to show any emotion, which makes it difficult to tell what he feels or what he's thinking. I had decided to nurse, so I took care of David almost exclusively. At first I think Bob was happy to have it that way, as he had never been exposed to a baby before and seemed nervous about it. Full-time caring for David put a terrific drain on me. I had more work to do during the day: more clothes to wash, the baby's room to finish, yard work, a part-time job, as well as David to care for. I began to grow more impatient with Bob because I got neither help nor sympathy nor understanding from him. All he could see was that because of David, I had less time for him.

When Bob did want to do more with David, such as put him to bed, David refused. He was more than happy to play with Daddy during the day, but when bedtime came, he wanted Mommy. This rejection must have hurt Bob and more strained feelings emerged in our relationship.

If David woke up with a nightmare or some discomfort during the night, I would lie down with him to make him feel safe and secure until he fell back to sleep. Sometimes, because I wasn't getting much sleep myself, I would fall asleep too. Bob became upset that I was sleeping with my son instead of him. I think that Bob wouldn't have objected as much if David had been a girl. He is jealous of David because our child takes so much of the time that I would normally have given him.

Bob isn't the only one who feels resentment: I do also. Bob comes home from work, buries himself in the paper and the mail, and gets perturbed if David distracts him. He fusses if David makes noise when he is trying to hear the news and the weather, and after dinner goes downstairs to listen to television undisturbed. Occasionally he plays with David and invites him to come downstairs. Usually I have to keep David busy and away from Bob and fix dinner at the same time. I have been with David all day long and I need a break. He needs his father. Instead, we get, "Shh, I can't hear the news."

When David was born I quit my job as a full-time employee to become a full-time mother, and that loss of additional income was hard to cope with. We were used to going out and getting whatever we wanted without hesitation and without thinking about the cost. My own wants changed, along with our new financial situation. I no longer desired new clothes, but I did want to buy clothes for David. Bob still saw things he wanted for himself and sometimes went ahead and bought them, leaving me to figure out how to budget them. Or he would complain about not being able to afford what he wanted. He resents the loss of income, and I feel he blames me and David for this problem. I, in turn, feel resentment toward Bob, both because I feel he should learn to spend more wisely and because I find myself wishing he wanted to do more for David.

I feel that bringing up a child properly is a full-time job and should be treated as such. I try to expose David to as much of the world as I can. During the summer I spend the days taking him to see people or outdoor things. This consumes most of my time, and it is harder to get my housework done. Bob comes home from work to a messy house, and David and I are outdoors playing in the lake or talking to the neighbors. He becomes angry and interrogates me: "I've worked very hard all day. What have you done?" What he doesn't realize is that answering our son's demands, providing stimulation and encouragement for him to learn and grow, is also hard work.

At one point I took on a part-time job to help with the money problem. It wasn't much and I could do it at home, but it turned out to be more than I could handle. I couldn't work while David was up; he was a busy boy and needed constant watching. I once left the room long enough to make a *short* phone call, and in that time he climbed up on the stove, turned on the burners, and burned his foot pretty badly; I was then blamed for not watching him more closely. So I had to wait to work until David napped. As the naps grew shorter and less frequent, I had to spend several evenings working after David had gone to bed. This bothered Bob because I was not devoting my full-time attention to him. It's not as if he were used to a close interaction between us because we didn't have that. Usually he watched television or fell asleep on the couch, but he needed the security of knowing that if he wanted me for anything, I would be there, ready to listen to him.

Once in a while he went to bed without me, but usually he stayed up waiting for me. He grumbled a great deal in either case, feeling that I should go to bed with him whether I was ready or not. This really bothered me; after all, I didn't want the job and had only taken it because he had made me feel I had to for the money. Finally I couldn't stand it any longer and quit the job. More resentment built up between Bob and me, and he placed even more blame on David.

Shortly after David's birth, I apparently went through some sort of physical or emotional change which to this day I cannot understand and am just now, after two years, starting to get over. The thought of having any sexual relation with Bob made me sick. I couldn't tell him because I feared he would be hurt and resent David even more. And how could I expect him to understand what

I didn't understand myself? I succumbed to his needs as often as I could stand it, which became less and less frequently. Each time was harder than the last, until I couldn't stand to have him touch me at all, for any reason. I felt as if I were being raped. Raped in the worst kind of way. I couldn't cry out or get away from it; I knew it would happen again; and I couldn't even talk to anyone about it. I began to hate and resent Bob for putting me through it, and I'm sure he was confused and angry with me. I found myself turning more toward my son because I knew that there I would find nothing but total friendship and love without any physical demands. And so, there was yet another problem to contend with between us — an unspoken but terrible one.

Having a baby is certainly more work than I thought it would be, although I love it and wouldn't give up motherhood for anything in the world. However, I wasn't prepared for the strain it has placed on my marriage.

ALICE JOHNSON is a pseudonym. The author and her family live in a country town.

New Challenges to the Relationship

JANE C. PEDERSEN

After attending our first Lamaze class, I thought that my relationship with my husband was doomed. Steve's simple statement, "There is no pain in childbirth," which followed the viewing of a childbirth film in which the woman in labor was obviously in pain, triggered off the most serious fight of our nine-year relationship. I was so angry at his absolute denial of reality, to say nothing of my own feelings and fears, that we did not speak for two days, something which had never before occurred.

I did not know how we could solve our communication problems. I was vaguely aware that Steve's denial meant that he himself was frightened and unprepared to handle the anticipated stress of my childbirth pain and possibly the entire pregnancy as well. But I could not help him. I was needy and unwilling to deal with his problems; after all, I was the one who was pregnant; I was the one who had to deliver the baby.

The fighting depressed me, and I found myself wondering what it would be like to raise this child alone, without Steve, since at times we seemed too far apart to be able to close the gap. I needed comfort, support, encouragement, and, above all, mothering; but Steve was obviously dealing with the pregnancy in his own way, and, like me, he was also having a difficult time giving.

Our relationship has always been characterized by a strong sense of independence and by the opportunity to be free to be our own person. Somewhere we were taught that to be needy, to give and be given to, to be comforting and to be comforted, depicts a weak self-image. Yet during my pregnancy I wished to be more dependent on Steve, without really knowing how to ask for what I wanted. Although Steve was excited about having a baby, it did not seem to consume his every waking moment. My increased demands and dependency caused Steve to distance himself from me. They also fostered communication problems which were not easily, if actually ever, resolved. I had anticipated that pregnancy, like parenting, would be a joint venture; that what I felt, Steve would share similarly; that somehow he too would be different. I think that if my own mother had been available to nurture and support me (she had died the year before), it would have lessened my high expectations of Steve. Part of me still hadn't finished resolving that loss. I hadn't finished being a child, yet I was about to assume the responsibility of motherhood. It was frightening.

───────────

After nine trying months of stress and disequilibrium in our relationship, the event of our lifetime finally happened. Suddenly, all the unsynchronized moments of our pregnancy vanished; we were again together. Our feelings meshed. One statement would trigger an abundant surging of energy, unlike anything we had ever experienced. It was better than orgasm — an incredible explosion of sensation, emotions, and feelings, and all because of one eight-pound-five-ounce baby boy. I remained in that euphoric, dream state for the whole week I was in the hospital. I could think of nothing but my baby and his father and the three of us as a new unit.

As the days of the first week went by, however, Steve had to fulfill his other responsibilities. He had to go to work, feed the cats, look at the bills, and think about whether there was enough gas in the car to get to the hospital. I had forgotten that he was in the "real world" and I was not. By the time we were ready to leave the hospital, I could not understand why he wouldn't drop everything and stay home for a few days with us until we adjusted to the routine and I recovered from the surgery. So, as delightful as our experience with the baby continued to be, only one week later there were new stresses on the relationship. Fortunately we coped much better with these "afterbirth" stresses than we had with those that occurred during our pregnancy. The presence of the baby somehow neutralized many of the negative feelings. Andrew had added a new dimension to our relationship and a new reason for our existence, both as individuals and as a married couple. It was impossible to ignore the joy we shared or to deny the bond that he had created between us.

Still, I can now understand why there are some marital situations where couples spend seemingly enjoyable years raising a family, only to find that afterward, there is little left in their relationship. Indeed, children can be a real communication distancer between a couple. In our brief time as parents, we rarely talk to each other about ourselves. Our conversation revolves around our shared joy with Andrew. We seldom have much eye contact because it is impossible to keep our eyes off our son. He is so beautiful, responsive, new, and visually stimulating; why would we want to look at each other when we have been doing that for nine years? If we want to maintain the quality of our relationship, we will obviously have to allocate specific time periods for ourselves, without interference from Andrew. But for the moment we are choosing not to do that; we still can't get enough of him.

Although Andrew is an easy child to be with, by late afternoon I feel worn out from having cared for a baby all day. When Steve walks in the door, I am grateful to have someone with whom to share the responsibility for this fragile being. And when Steve doesn't come home at five because he has to work late, I feel terribly angry. I worry that their relationship won't be as strong as Andrew's and mine because I spend so much more time with our child.

I find myself wishing that Steve would value my new role as mother more, and that he would praise me as he used to when I was in the work world. Although I think I am a fairly good mother, I need some reassurance. I am also having difficulty with my new role as a "housewife." I would like my house to be clean and tidy, but unfortunately it never meets my standards. So I feel like a failure at homemaking, which should be such a simple job. Sometimes I'm not smiling and cheerful when Steve comes home, the way the movies or television portray stay-at-home women, and I feel guilty about that. When Steve buries his head in the newspaper and "ignores" me, I become resentful. Yet I wonder what I have to talk about that would be of interest besides the baby.

In these five brief months since Andrew's birth, the adjustments that Steve and I have had to make as individuals and as a couple have been challenging. I often think of the future with pleasure because of Andrew. But I wonder too how our marriage will change during those years. When we are again only two, will our relationship have withstood the stress?

JANE C. PEDERSEN is a psychiatric social worker who practices part-time in Chicago. Her son was born shortly before her thirty-fourth birthday.

8

Redefining Relationships:
Mother

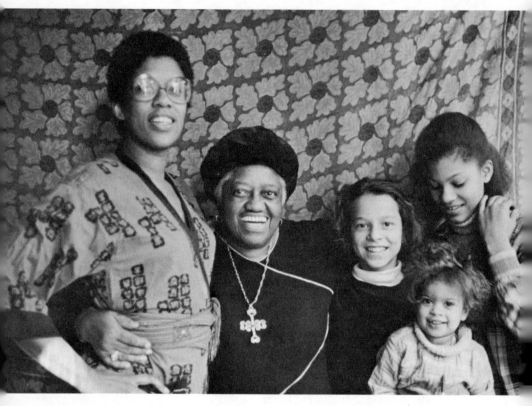

Melissa Shook

Mother Love

MYRNA FINN

My first vivid recollection of the love my mother and I shared is of a summer vacation when I was about four years old. We were playing a game which we called "Mumpty." My mother would tickle my belly and my neck, especially under my chin, and say "Mumpty." I would then squeal with delight. We would laugh, kiss, and hug one another joyfully. The game had no particular rules; we played it only when we were alone. It became our special way of expressing our love for one another.

Another clear memory is of me as a seven-year-old telling my mother that I wished I could cut off her head, take it to school with me, and put it on my desk so I could kiss her all day. Although it may sound macabre, she was touched by the feelings and sentiment behind my little fantasy, and she still reminds me of it today.

In my early years, my love for my mother was total and all-encompassing. She appreciated, delighted, and reveled in my love, while I grew, developed, and thrived on her love for me.

During my late adolescence and early twenties, however, I began to resist and detest my mother's love, feeling encumbered, consumed, and oppressed by it. At that time I entered into a stage of redefining my identity. In order to assert my independence, I found it necessary to isolate myself from my personal history as if I had arrived on the planet as a free-floating and fully grown adult. I convinced myself that if I wanted to succeed as a responsible, capable adult, my mother's love was not only unimportant, but would be a barrier to my achieving "personhood."

I was not living at home at this point. Indeed, I had left my homeland (Canada) and fled to the United States to create a new life for myself. I had rejected my mother, and I told her very little of what was going on in my life. I was operating on the premise that if I let her know anything about me, somehow she could control me; if I accepted her love, I was subject to her values and lifestyle. In order to establish my own identity and power, I needed to reject both her and her love.

As I began to know, like, and feel comfortable with myself, it became easier to accept and appreciate my mother's love. It became natural once again to say, "I love you" to my mother. My subsequent marriage only strengthened this renewed bond with her.

───────────

When I became pregnant, I realized that I wanted my mother with me very soon after the delivery to mother, nurture, and care for me. This desire surprised me: I had not needed my mother for years, and suddenly, as I was on the verge of motherhood, my desire for her care and nurturing reemerged. I even considered having her present at the birth, both to share this intimacy with her and to help compensate for past omissions. My husband and I finally decided against it. However, to this day part of me wishes she had been present.

So I did the next best thing: I requested that my mother take care of me as soon as I came home from the hospital. She was thrilled to be asked and stayed for two weeks. She not only took care of the house, meals, me, and my son, but she showed me how to do the "little things" that only a mother knows to make Jed more comfortable. She was a tremendous support in those shaky, scary, and exhausting early weeks.

Each time I responded to my son's cries to be nursed, no matter what the hour, she would wake up with me to bring me water, help change diapers, and keep me company. She followed this routine with me for her entire two-week stay. During the days, she would read to me from books on child care. She even came along to the pediatrician for the second-week checkup to help ask the right questions, and to be certain that all was perfect with her new grandson. She was as involved with him as I was, and as close to me as she had ever been.

During those weeks together, our relationship changed dramatically. We were both mothers. This meant that we were, in a real sense, equals. For the first time, I could begin to understand a mother's love for her child, and therefore my mother's love for me. I could share with my mother the great depth and breadth of feelings that arise when one gives birth to a child and sees that child grow and develop. I began to understand how a mother's heart warms and glows as she watches her child achieve or laugh with glee. I sensed how a mother suffers when her child is hurt, frightened, or unhappy. As a nonparent, I had heard the words and intellectualized the feelings; but as a mother, I could *feel* the experience. Now we are both givers of maternal love rather than one a giver and one a recipient. We share this giving and are bound closer together by it. I love this new connection with my mother, and I am grateful that motherhood has enabled me to experience it.

I feel truly fulfilled as a woman since giving birth and becoming a mother. And since I have become a mother, I feel that my mother accepts and respects me more because I have fulfilled one of the cultural norms. Her joy and support, her encouragement and strong personal feelings about children and family life, lead me to believe that she is very proud that I have become a mother.

When my mother left me after those first two weeks, I felt as if the world were coming to an end. Although she had to return home and I needed to learn to take care of my child, I felt abandoned, frightened, and lonely. During her stay, she had been my mom who could do no wrong, and I had been her little girl once again. Suddenly I had to be grown up. It was a tearful, sorrowful departure, like losing my best friend. Part of the sadness was my fear of having to do it alone. Part was the loss of the intimacy I had shared with my mother during those weeks.

Her visit left an indelible mark on our relationship. We speak to and see each other more frequently than ever. She is intensely interested in knowing all about her grandson. She relishes each and every detail I provide, both about him and about me in my role as mother. I delight in sharing these things with her — as if to compensate for all the intimacy and intricate details which I didn't share with her as an adolescent and young adult.

My relationship with my mother since I became a mother has changed most in that I am now willing and able to give her unconditional love. Although we are very different from one another, varying widely in our likes and dislikes, lifestyles and values, our love transcends these differences. Her example has helped me to give my love freely and totally to my son. His birth has enabled me to do the same with my mother.

MYRNA FINN was born in Montreal, Canada, and left home when she turned twenty-one to pursue a career in communications disorders. She obtained her doctorate from Boston University and lives in Brookline, Massachusetts.

My Mother's Ghost

JANE WATS

"Do you ever find yourself sounding like your mother when you talk to Emily?" I asked a friend as we sat watching our two-year-olds play. "As a matter of fact, yes," she replied, "and it used to make me uneasy. But it doesn't bother me in the least now. I realize that I like my mother's product." Nothing could have made me feel worse. My friend's sanguine response added another dimension to the anxiety plaguing me since my sixth month of pregnancy. Not only was I doomed to resemble my mother and to relive her life — something I had been trying to avoid since adolescence — but my child would suffer as a result. Inevitably, he too would come to dislike his mother's product.

I hadn't always felt this way about my mother. As a child I had engaged in rich fantasies of mothering. My favorite toy until I was ten had been a "Blessed Event" doll, a life-sized replica of a newborn infant. And I remember, when I was four, watching my mother with awe as she cared for my baby brother. In my impatience to have a child of my own, I would often put on one of my mother's dresses, stuff it with pillows, and pretend that I was pregnant.

When I reached adolescence my attitude toward my mother changed. My brother had become "difficult," an underachiever and disciplinary problem in school and a disruptive member of the family at home, riddling our lives with constant outbursts. As I observed my mother struggling — and failing — with my brother, I began to question her competence, first as a child rearer and then as a human being.

Aside from her husband and children, my mother had no interests, no life of her own. Some women belonged to clubs, played bridge, joined the PTA, or did volunteer work at the local hospital. Others read books or took classes at the local college. Some even returned to school to finish bachelor degrees or to do graduate work. My mother did none of these. She had no real circle of friends. Nor did she seem interested in life beyond the pale of our family. At dinnertime, she engaged less and less frequently in discussions. And when she did, her remarks struck me as highly subjective and emotional. By the time I was fifteen, I no longer admired her in any way. In fact, I consciously set out to become her antithesis.

For a while, all went well. I attended a prestigious Ivy League college, graduated with full honors, and easily completed my doctorate in French literature. Both my parents were extremely proud of my accomplishments, and time away from home gradually obscured my deeper feelings toward my mother. By the time I married a fellow graduate student, I had achieved a strong identity of my own and looked forward to a successful career and fulfilling life. Unfortunately, however, because of the tightness of the job market for Ph.D.'s, I was soon faced with joblessness in the small university town where my husband had found a teaching position. I spent several frantic months pursuing every conceivable angle on the job market. And for the first time in many years, I was troubled by visions of my mother's empty life. I began to feel that her inability to find fulfillment might also be my fate.

Even a job as copywriter for the university press did not dispel my fears. I wanted desperately to teach at the college level, and there were definitely no possibilities in the town or its surroundings. The only thing to do, my husband and I finally concurred, was for me to look for a job nationally and to relocate, as a couple, wherever I could find a suitable position. Since Bob was more marketable, he was most likely to find a job wherever we settled down. In the meantime, since Bob's contract did not expire for over a year, we decided to have a child.

For the first five months of my pregnancy, I was euphoric.

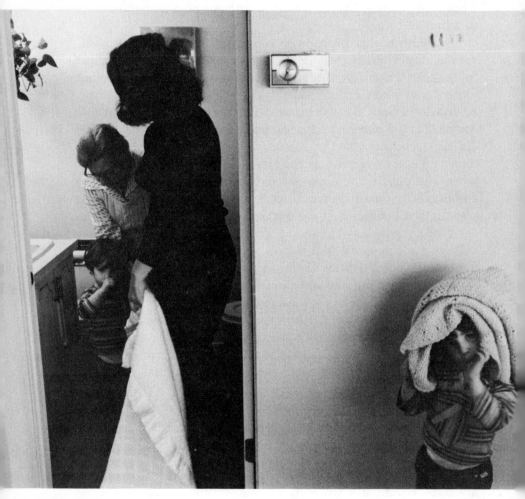

Gail LeBoff

Never had I felt better or more in harmony with myself. Then, one day as I sat having lunch with old friends, I felt the baby kicking and I panicked. Shaken, I tried to discover the reasons for my uncharacteristic reaction. Usually I relished every movement of the baby, luxuriating in my ability to nurture the life inside me and in the intimacy I already sensed with my future child. What had happened? As the weeks wore on and my attacks of anxiety increased, old feelings about my mother, along with suspicions of my own inadequacy, surfaced. The blueprint for my life that I had so carefully drawn during adolescence had failed to become a reality. After all, I had not yet begun the career for which I had so carefully prepared, and I was about to have a baby. What was to ensure me that the situation would change in the future? Gradually I was overcome with feelings of helplessness and hopelessness. If my mother's life was a failure, mine would be too.

When several months later I gave birth to a beautiful baby boy, the obstetrician said that he had never, in his twenty-five years of practice, seen a mother so relieved at her baby's good bill of health. "I just can't understand your reaction. There was no reason to suspect any problems," he told me as I tearfully cradled my wide-eyed son minutes after his birth. What the doctor didn't know was that for the last months of my pregnancy, my feelings of inadequacy had been translated into an obsessive fear that my baby would be malformed. In addition to my relief at my baby's good health, my elation had another source. My first-born was a son, while my mother's had been a girl. Certainly, I thought, this was a sign that from now on my life would be very different from hers.

My elation continued while I remained in the hospital. But when I returned home, I became depressed. My mother had come to care for me, and upon seeing her, I immediately remembered my months of anxiety at the end of my pregnancy. Also, she seemed uncomfortable, hesitant about doing even the simplest of household chores, and fearful of handling her new grandson. I had to help her prepare all the meals since even the prospect of baking a chicken overwhelmed her. She too was depressed, and her presence only created new tensions for my husband and me. To make matters worse, within several days my previously peaceful son began showing definite signs of colic. Suddenly I was gripped by yet another fear: like my brother, my child would be "difficult." For the first time in my life, I understood my mother's heartbreak as she groped for ways to deal with my brother and his problems. Yet instead of sympathy, I experienced only rage, blaming my mother for my problems also. When she left after a week of cold war, I was thrilled to see her go.

Over the next few weeks, as I accustomed myself to caring for my baby, I settled into a state of mild depression. I forced myself to think only about the present: nursing; relieving the symptoms of colic; sharing motherhood with friends. My mother phoned often, but my husband usually supplied alibis so that I didn't have to talk to her. "She's nursing; she's resting," or, "She's just run to the store for some milk," he would say. My mother seemed to accept his pro forma excuses, never asking me to call back or questioning him about the exact state of my health. And on those rare occasions when I did speak with her, I tried to remain as detached and impersonal as possible. I would even pretend that she was not, in fact, my mother, but simply a friend interested in my well-being and that of my baby. My strategies worked well for a while, until my husband was unexpectedly offered a teaching position that would require another move. After days of emotionally charged discussion and much soul-searching on both our parts, we accepted it. I was in no condition, we decided, to begin a job hunt of my own. Also, we had previously lived happily in that particular city, and had many friends there. We both thought that the move would brighten my state of mind. I would remain home for one year with our son, and then certainly I would be able to find a job at one of the many colleges in the area.

Things went according to plan. We bought a small frame home (which in no way resembled my parents'), and I began canvassing the area colleges for teaching possibilities. I accepted a part-time position with a small liberal arts college, and as I slowly regained my self-confidence, I was gradually able to relate to my mother again. My success at interviewing and securing a job delivered me — if only temporarily — from the fear of walking in her footsteps. Once I began to behave more cordially, my mother was able to establish a warm relationship with her grandson. I came to look forward to her visits and enjoyed sharing my adorable baby's triumphs with her. Finally I was able to look at her and think, "She is my mother and I love her." However, I was always quick to add, "But my life will be nothing like hers."

By the second semester of teaching I was physically and emotionally exhausted. The college insisted on the total devotion of its faculty: in the classroom, on committees, and during extracurricular and social events. The students seemed to make excessive demands, and I had two new courses to prepare each term, as well as a husband and an active, gravity-defying toddler to care for at home. I began to feel out of control, unable to function well in *any* of my roles. I despaired of achieving any success in my career. Once again my old fears reappeared, this time with a vengeance. I was certain that no matter what I did, I would become my mother, that my life would ineluctably lead to endless days of house cleaning, soap operas, and solitude. What was more, my two-year-old began acting his age, insisting on having his own way, refusing to do anything his father or I wanted. He was difficult. He reminded me of my brother.

At the same time my mother, perhaps coincidentally, perhaps for well-founded reasons, became highly critical of both me and her grandson. "How can you be a good mother when you are so exhausted by your job? A mother should be at home with her child," she would say icily over the telephone. During visits she commented that I made too much of a fuss over my son, that I touched and kissed him too frequently. And when he misbehaved, even mildly, she would say, "He's always been difficult. Remember his terrible colic!"

Whether consciously or not, my mother seemed to be conspiring against my mental well-being. By the end of the year I was profoundly depressed, and I began paying biweekly visits to a psychiatrist. A compassionate and highly intelligent person, he helped ease me through the next two years. With his support, I was able to continue teaching and to gain more confidence in myself both as an individual and as a mother. I was able to relax more and more with my son. We became fine companions. Relations with my mother, however, worsened. Unable to penetrate my newly shored defenses, she turned to her grandson, often expressing overt hostility toward him, reprimanding him for the slightest infraction of her rules of good conduct and rebuffing his sincere efforts at reconciliation. After one especially unhappy visit, I was forced to tell my father (I dreaded direct confrontations) that my mother was no longer a welcome guest in my home.

I have not seen my mother for ten months. Although I am now wise enough to abstain from predictions about the future, I do look forward to my mother's imminent visit to my home, confident that my four-year-old is a wonderful child and beginning to believe that I am my own person, no longer merely my mother's ghost.

JANE WATS is the pseudonym of a French teacher who lives in the western part of the country.

9

Redefining Relationships:
Friends

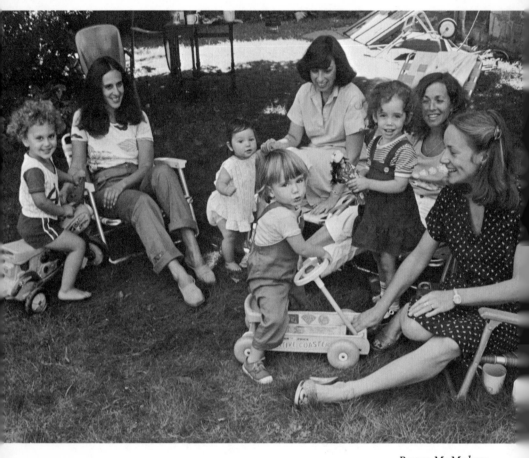

Peggy McMahon

Thoughts on Friendship and Feminism

SARAH D. PICK

I am a relatively young mother, and although I don't see mother-hood and feminism as being necessarily incompatible, my feminist friends do. For me, the hardest emotional adjustment after Daniel's birth has not been with my husband or parents, but with my non-mother friends.

Within my small circle of friends, a mother at twenty-four seems quite young. (Ten years ago, it would have seemed quite old.) I understand their wariness over the baby and my motherhood: they are faced with so much societal/familial/media pressure to "settle down" that women who feel that this lifestyle is not of their choosing become defensive toward anything family oriented. The very act of having a baby seems to imply certain political beliefs, and I am viewed as being party to the pressure on single women, whatever my own beliefs may be. It takes a lot of subtle reassuring on my part to remind friends that while having a baby is what Joe and I wanted to do now, I am not advocating that they do likewise.

I try to understand my friends' negative reactions to my moth-erhood, but I would like some understanding myself. It hurts me when friends are not able to support this major change in my life. I'm not saying that they should become mothers also, but I don't intend to feel guilty for choosing to become a mother because they aren't ready to deal with it.

Although I am usually very confident and self-assured, new motherhood was a period of time when I needed constant reassurance. I wanted to hear others tell me that all babies cry, or that Daniel was getting enough milk. What I did not feel like discussing was how Joe and I were sharing baby care, and how many times a day Joe changed the baby's diaper. It's not that the partner's sharing of baby care is not important — it is. But what I needed was nurturing from those friends, or at least some encouragement.

Looking back, I can see that the kind of advice I needed almost had to come from other mothers. Pregnancy, labor, and the early days of motherhood are events that you can only comprehend totally when you experience them yourself.

As a new mother, I feel in some ways as if I have joined a new club. I can sit and discuss baby products and behavior for hours with women I would not necessarily have had much in common with before. For me, one of the most positive aspects of motherhood is that it is something shared *only* by women. Motherhood brings women together, to some degree breaking down racial and social barriers. This itself is a feminist goal, even if certain feminists downplay motherhood because it has been used against them. We do not, however, need to reject motherhood. We merely have to expand the traditional view of it.

A long-time resident of Baltimore, Maryland, SARAH D. PICK plans to work at a hospital lab when her son turns one. She is currently taking a medical technician's course and a class in carpentry.

New Feelings About Old Friends

MARY PAINTER BOHLEN

Soon after the birth of my son, colleagues from work — newspaper people — began stopping by the house. Some were so interested in the baby that they had little time to talk to me. Surprisingly, I was not jealous because I too was focusing on the baby. Others, however, attempted to carry on work-as-usual conversations, virtually ignoring the fact that little Will was around.

And now, five months after Will's arrival, the realization that my relationship with those work friends will never be the same has hit me with full force.

While most of my childless friends have been accepting of the changes in me and are interested in Will's development, a few have continued to pretend that he doesn't exist. They almost never ask about him and seem to resent any time I must devote to him. A very few go so far as to welcome any complaint I might express about motherhood, as if encouraging me to talk about the negative side and thus prove I miss my old life. This pulls me in opposite directions: I feel glad they still care about me as a person, yet unhappy they can't accept my life's newest turn.

Sometimes I enjoy the way motherhood has changed my friendships. I now have a new life to share — a life most of my single, working friends find foreign and therefore intriguing. It is as if watching a new person develop opens their often cynical reporters' eyes to life anew. Often they regard Will with wonder and transfer some of that to me for having helped bring him into the world.

Other times, though, the change in our relationship saddens me. Gone, at least for now and perhaps forever, are the casual after-work get-togethers, the lingering over drinks or coffee, discussing the latest political struggles, the coziness of sharing an early morning legislative session while the rest of the city sleeps. If I keep turning down their invitations to go out for a drink because I want to get home to see Will, will they stop asking?

Along with changes in my relationship with long-time childless friends is a shift in dealing with other parents. So long as I was working and surrounded mostly by childless co-workers, I had little time to develop friendships with other parents. Now I seem to seek out other mothers, and they me, as if we are drawn together by a mutual need to share the experience. Sometimes we exchange information on the most mundane aspects of child rearing, but often we lean on each other for support. With other mothers I can be negative about motherhood without running the risk of making someone think I don't like the overall experience. Or I can be positive without sounding as if I'm trying to convince someone to become a parent, too.

I find that I am now much more selfish with my time — something I suspect will become even stronger when I return to work. When I accept an invitation to go out, I try to get as much enjoyment out of it as possible. I don't take total freedom or time for granted anymore. When I have time for only one telephone call before Will's lunch, I am selective about whom I call. More often than not, it will be another mother. But it also is nice to have friends I can call when I *don't* feel like discussing parenting at all.

No matter what I am doing, I know that always, in the back of my mind, I'll stop and wonder what Will is doing — if he is safe and happy and full. I've acquired that typical parental trait of scattered attention, the need to keep one eye on a busy child while trying to focus on an adult conversation, and not doing either very well. My friends sense this, and I imagine that it makes them more reluctant to share what is going on in their lives with me.

In spite of the difficulties, motherhood — with its deep emotional ties to another person — has made me value my emotional ties to friends. I appreciate their support of the change in my life and I try to be sensitive to the changes in theirs. Seeing life through the eyes of a small child as he or she discovers the world seems to help an adult look for the beauty and wonder in all things, especially other people.

MARY PAINTER BOHLEN continued working as a state government and political reporter for United Press International in Springfield, Illinois, until a week before her due date. After a maternity leave, she plans — not without some mixed feelings — to return to UPI full time.

The Competitive Sport of Mothering

CAROLYN HARDY JENSEN

I had always assumed that when the urge to compete was passed out, I was passed over. Whether it was a simple card game or a piano contest, I usually wanted to do the best I was capable of, but unlike many of my friends, I never had a strong desire to win or to be "number one."

Then along came motherhood. When it was first confirmed

that a new life was indeed growing inside me, I felt pure joy. My concerns revolved only around me, my baby, my husband, and the grandparents-to-be. I never dreamed that other mothers and their children were to play such a large part in how I felt about *my* child and myself as a mother.

I think my competitive feelings first appeared during a conversation with my own mother when I was six-months pregnant with my first child. We were both excited about the baby, her first grandchild. I happened to mention that I had purchased an orthodontic pacifier for the baby, and instead of complimenting me on having the good judgment to protect my baby's future teeth, my mother insisted that my baby would not need such a thing. The reason? Neither of her two children had required one. As a result of our conversation, I felt that if I used the pacifier, it would mean that my baby was inferior to her children, or at least she might think so. And that's when I began to compete — wanting praise for both my child and my mothering.

I was amazed that *I* could possess such strong feelings about wanting a child to be just as good as or better than someone else's — even my mother's — when the child wasn't even born yet! Where did these feelings come from? Could I bear it if my child turned out to be below average?

One of my most painful experiences as a mother happened at a morning coffee for five women and their young children, all under four years. My two-year-old threw a wild tantrum when another child took away her cup of juice. I could not leave, because someone else had given me a ride, so I tried to remain calm while everyone witnessed my daughter's antisocial behavior.

For days afterward I was ill from anger and shame: anger at the other child's mother for not making her boy give back the cup; and anger at the other three mothers for silently witnessing such a display and for judging me (at least I thought they were). I was ashamed that I had allowed the situation to develop. And I was ashamed of my innocent daughter for not being the best-behaved child at the get-together.

Studies indicate that parents use much more physical forms of punishment when in the presence of outsiders than they do in the privacy of their home. I find myself reacting more strongly in public because I want people to think I'm a superior parent who can control my child.

I find it easier to cultivate a friendship with another mother when my children (or a friend's) are not present because I am freed from concern about whether my child will behave as well as the others. I don't have to worry that my child might scratch a baby's face or break a glass vase; I need not fear that the other mother will judge me.

My friends and I often compare the physical development of our children, as when they learned to crawl or walk, or when a tooth came in. If my child is slow in these areas, it does not bother me. I only compete in the areas for which the mother is solely responsible — areas which require teaching — such as potty-training or control of aggression. If mine is behind in these areas, I resent being judged; and if it's someone else's child that I am witnessing, I feel sorry for the other mother, even while I may be judging her.

About the most uncomforting remark a mother can make to me when I mention a problem with my daughter is, "My child never did that." It makes me wonder just how I can be so inadequate as to be the only one confronted with the particular issue. It's so refreshing when another mother relates some of her difficulties with her children.

It's a common complaint from mothers that nonmothers have no business giving advice about child rearing. Frankly, I'd rather be criticized by a person without children (over whom I feel some authority) than by another mother who has "walked in my shoes."

After five years of mothering, I am trying to take competition less seriously. I think that having more than one child helps change the "needing baby to be perfect" attitude, perhaps because I don't have as much time to dwell on the accomplishments or failures of the "one and only." Also, with two children, if my one child is misbehaving chances are pretty good that my other child is not causing any problems. Having my second child has also made me much less critical of other mothers. I realize that all children are not alike, that some are simply more difficult to raise.

CAROLYN HARDY JENSEN lives in Mt. Pleasant, Iowa, with her husband of nine years and her two children.

10

---

*Sexuality
and Motherhood*

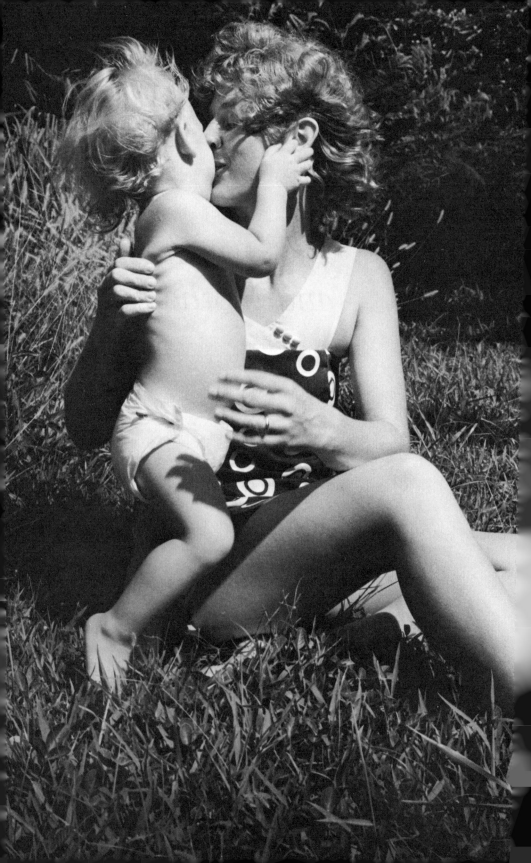

Mothertalk

A GROUP DISCUSSION ON SEXUALITY AND MOTHERHOOD

Sexual Feelings During and After Pregnancy

BETH: As soon as I learned that I was pregnant, I identified myself as a pregnant woman, not a sexual one. I gained forty pounds, and I didn't care. I loved looking and feeling pregnant. Even as a new mother, I felt fine being fat. I was a nursing mother, and my breasts were enormous. I didn't care what I looked like. Michael and I hardly had sex at all when I was pregnant — in fact, hardly at all for the first year. Only very gradually did I regain my desire to have sex, and it seemed like he wasn't interested in sex either.

RACHEL: What bothered me was the sense of loss of control. Sex to me meant milk spurting out, loss of vaginal muscle control, loss of control over my whole body. I hated the fact that we couldn't have sex in the morning, or before tea in the evening. Suddenly, sex was possible only at night, so that even timing was out of my control. But I was too tired at night; I had to get back in shape; and I basically felt that I was not myself.

SARAH: I didn't feel attractive the first few months after birth. I didn't feel sexy to men, or to my husband. I had huge breasts that were not characteristic of me. If Ruth cried, we would have to jump up and that was the end of lovemaking. It took a long time to get back to normal sexuality for me and for Thomas. Ruth was the center of our lives.

LORRAINE: Two weeks after our son's birth, we visited the gynecologist. Robert asked if we could make love, or if we had to wait even longer. The doctor told him to ask me. *I* certainly felt ready! Look, we're very sexual and remained so all during my pregnancy. In fact, we made love until the day before I gave birth. I can't really relate to all of your nonsexual feelings.

LESLIE: I was also sexually active during pregnancy. I found it to be a tremendous turn-on. The different positions required while being quite pregnant were arousing to me. I loved feeling the changes in my body. I have big hips, and when my breasts became large with milk, my hips suddenly looked rather small by comparison. I never before had so much confidence in my body. Everything female in me was working for the first time in my life. Pregnancy, labor, postpartum period — they had gone smoothly, and left me feeling womanly. I bought new clothes and felt positive about being a new mother, and an attractive woman.

CANDY: I loved being pregnant but did not feel sexy. And even after the birth, for me, motherhood and sexuality did not go together. But I frankly didn't care because all of my life energy was going into mothering. It took us a good year to get back to our sexual lives, and now we have a stronger sexual relationship than ever before. Sexuality and motherhood have finally merged, but it was a long time in coming.

ANNE: After my Caesarean section and the disappointment of not giving birth vaginally, I almost felt like a virgin. I experienced that same tightness, and it hurt me to have sex. I even started to dread it because I was afraid of the pain. Long after I should have felt fine, I had this problem. There always seemed to be a burning sensation and pressure. Clearly I was having psychological reactions to having had a Caesarean. After a year, I remember crying because sex was actually okay — not great — once. I can't tell you how long sex was stressful to me.

Sexual Feelings Our Children Have

LESLIE: Matthew is almost four and is definitely going through the oedipal stage. He wants to kiss me on my mouth. If I'm lying down, he will come into the bed and announce that he is going to get in on Daddy's side. He'll get into hugging and kissing me — not petting, of course, but pretty intense. Sometimes when John comes home, Matthew slams the door on him and screams that he wants John out of the room.

ANNE: How does John react?

LESLIE: Well, John is tired at the end of the day and the last thing he wants is to walk into the house and have someone screaming at him to leave. He tried to put an end to it, although he doesn't want to overreact either. We both know it's a natural, necessary stage. Still, it's difficult when Matthew has fantasies about having made a baby because we had read him a book earlier about how babies are made. Or when he gets into exposing himself. He started pulling out his penis and laughing, saying, "Hey, look at me!"

BETH: How do you respond? What do you do?

LESLIE: Sometimes I'll praise his body and say something about how nice *each* part is, including the penis.

CANDY: Do you ever get turned on?

LESLIE: No, but I worry that Matthew does. I enjoy hugging him in a motherly kind of way, but I do think it turns him on so I've become a little uncomfortable. I sometimes think that I shouldn't be so close to him.

CANDY: Is it because he gets an erection?

LESLIE: Yes. He once asked John to rub his penis. John said no but told him that he could rub it himself if it felt good, but that it was something private. Matthew became rather annoyed and said, "But Jane rubs it in day care." A few months younger than Matthew, Jane must have been fascinated by Matthew's erection.

SARAH: Ruth loves to be nude. I think that it's perfectly fine to run around the house nude at two, but I don't know how I'll feel about it when she's older.

RACHEL: Ruth takes baths with her father, doesn't she?

SARAH: Yes, but I don't think it's related to sexual feelings at all. It's a special time between her and Thomas — his time for taking care of her and relaxing with her. Ruth loves it, and I don't think that Thomas is ready to give it up either. They are having a good time together. He spends so little time with her; I would hate to see it end.

BETH: I think that Thomas should give up the bath with her soon. The longer it goes on, the harder it is going to be for Ruth. It's inappropriately arousing for a toddler to be bathing with her father.

LESLIE: When Matthew was two, I used to take baths with him. It eventually became clear to me that it was, indeed, inappropriate for me to bathe with him any longer. After the bath, he would act hostile to John, and he would become excited and confused.

ANNE: You mentioned that Matthew knew about how babies were made. Don't you think that he's too young to understand?

LESLIE: I only showed him the part of the book about how the infant grows inside the mother, and how it is born. I also told

159

him about sex differences between males and females. But I never read him the description on intercourse. He seemed able to handle those parts that we chose to read to him.

BETH: My feeling is that if sexual questions come up, never lie to your child. But offer as little information as they are willing to accept. At their young ages, I don't believe in giving too much incomprehensible information.

SARAH: The other day, Ruth asked me how the new baby is going to come out. It caught me unaware, and I didn't have time to think of a good explanation. Later, of course, I thought of a million great things to say to her. At the time, I was a bit shocked.

CANDY: Does Ruth play with herself? I know that very young boys do, but Dora is two, and I haven't noticed her doing it at all.

SARAH: Yes, Ruth masturbates frequently. I would like to bring up another issue. I've taught Ruth that I need my privacy when going to the bathroom. Thomas couldn't care less if she comes in and watches him, but I really do not want anyone — including my daughter — in the bathroom when I'm in there.

ANNE: A psychiatrist friend of mine said that he felt an enormous number of future problems stem from sexuality, and that it is very important to be modest. He thinks that you should close the door whenever you go to the bathroom. He said that kids become terrified when they see genitals bigger than their own, and that all that pubic hair can look frightening.

CANDY: Well, I don't close the bathroom door for anyone so why should I do it with Dora? Don't I have to be myself with her?

BETH: Aaron likes to crawl into bed with us sometimes, and Michael doesn't sleep with pajamas on. I told Michael that I don't feel so great about his being there naked with Aaron climbing over him. Sometimes Michael has an erection before he has urinated in the morning. So there he is with this hard-on, and Aaron comes in. I wish Michael would sleep with something on, but he won't.

CANDY: Neither of us sleeps with pajamas in the summer. Are you saying that we should change into clothes and be uncomfortable for the sake of our child?

BETH: Yes, as she gets older. Yes, I think so.

MARSHA: I would like to raise the issue of jealousy. When David and I are kissing, Steve gets upset. The minute we start hugging, we can feel his little hands between our legs to separate us. If he's brought into the action, then he's okay about it. When he was younger, it didn't bother him. Now he either wants to be hugged and kissed too, or for us not to do it at all.

BETH: They want to break us up, but they really don't want to. In my case, there's something else. Unlike most of your children, Aaron often prefers his father to me. In the night, he sometimes calls for him; he wants him. It hurts. Most kids call for their mother, but not Aaron.

CANDY: I feel terrible when Dora tells her father that he can't do this or that with her, that only Mommy can do it. I don't feel at all flattered. I feel bad that she can't relate to us both equally.

Sensuality

MARSHA: I find myself loving to touch Steve and feeling paranoid about it. He's not even two, so I tell myself that for a certain amount of months it's still all right for me to touch him. I love feeling his body, even touching his cute little genitals. Is that wrong?

RACHEL: I adore stroking and dancing with Elaine. She seems very sensual herself so I am just responding to her.

MARSHA: Yes, but she's a girl. I'm talking about touching Steve's genitals.

RACHEL: If you kiss him everywhere and leave a little patch untouched, you are giving him a message. If you touch him in a normal activity — diapering or cuddling — nothing is wrong with it.

MARSHA: I guess that I want to play with him but am afraid to, and stop myself. I don't want to cause him any sexual hang-up, but it's so wonderful loving his sweet little body. I also love long kisses with him.

LORRAINE: Marsha, you want to ravage Steve because you're so madly in love with your son. We all know that feeling.

CANDY: And what if there are undertones of sexuality? Is that so terrible? I would rather have those feelings to deal with than uptight restrictions.

SUSAN: Holding Ruth next to me when she's come out of a shower is a sensual delight. I can't say that it really turns me on, but it's lovely to have her naked body next to my skin.

LORRAINE: Our kids are growing up in such a different climate than we did. The vibrations are much more open. Imagine our mothers having a talk like this? I can't possibly imagine it.

CANDY: On the other hand, imagine our kids having a talk like this. I guess I'm not ready for that either.

MOTHERTALK is a group of new mothers who have been meeting monthly to discuss ways of dealing emotionally with certain issues raised by motherhood. Sometimes the meetings are animated and illuminating, but even when they are not, it is comforting and relaxing to sit around — without children or husbands — and feel the connectedness of being with other mothers.

Coping with Lesbianism and Motherhood

NADIA

I didn't know that I was a lesbian when I got married. I had very much wanted to be a mother, and I had assumed that a husband and a home had to go along with being one. It had never occurred to me to have female lovers. I had never had a relationship with a woman, and I didn't even know that lesbians existed. I knew about male homosexuals, but I just didn't think women did that kind of thing.

I was miserable in my marriage. For about ninety percent of the time, I was in therapy trying to figure out why I was so miserable. A lot of the problem, of course, was total sexual incompatibility. I hated sex. I avoided it as much as I could, yet hated myself for not being normal. I thought that I was frigid.

My first attraction to a woman in a physical way occurred

about a year before I became pregnant, but I was too frightened to act on my feelings, too frightened to find out if they were real.

I was already a mother (Abel was a little over a year old), and my husband was away for the weekend, when I had my first lesbian relationship. I went to a Halloween dance with the woman. When we came back we just fell into making love. I remember thinking, No wonder sex with men is so bad! Being with a woman was fantastic, even though I had misgivings about her as a person (she was unstable and I couldn't count on her for anything).

The next day, when my husband came home, I ran up to him and announced that the most fabulous thing had happened to me. Then I told him all about my experience. I assumed that he would want to know that I was able to enjoy sex at last. Of course, his response was anger, rejection, and jealousy. He couldn't believe that I would tell him about it; I guess he saw a lot more in it than even I did. I think he realized that since I had never felt that way about sex with him, our relationship and marriage were doomed. I, on the other hand, was so caught up in finally understanding what had been wrong with me sexually that I was blind to what it meant for the future of our marriage.

It was well over a year and a half before we finally separated. For a long time, I rejected the idea; I recognized that I was attracted to women physically, but I believed that a relationship could not be built on physical attraction alone, and that children could not be raised outside of a heterosexual marriage. I hoped that we could stay married and I could have lesbian relationships on the side. That way Abel would be taken care of and have two parents, yet I could satisfy my sexual needs.

I went through a lot of self-hatred about my sexual feelings; I felt that being a mother was primary, and that my sexual needs would have to be put aside. It was a very hard time for me. I certainly did not know any lesbians who were also mothers, and I could not conceive of sustaining a child within a lesbian relationship. I opted to stay in my marriage and put off dealing with my lesbianism.

Much later, when I finally started going to a gay center, I met women who never mentioned anything about being mothers, or wanting to be. I didn't think, in fact, that there was such a thing as a lesbian mother. I thought I was a freak.

Eventually I met a woman who was a mother, and we started a relationship. I happened to meet her the day that I was moving into my own apartment, since I had decided I needed time alone in order to figure out what I was going to do with my life. It was so exciting to me that the woman I met was both a mother and a lesbian. Looking back, I see that I fell in love with an image, rather than with a person. One of the reasons the relationship ended was because we disagreed over our mothering. It was a major source of our arguments. I had a dream that we would share our child responsibilities and build a family unit together, but she did not want to. She wanted the children to be incidental, and I could never accept that.

By then I had left my marriage, and there was no going back. And I had at last accepted my lesbianism. I discovered, much to my surprise, that there were other lesbians who were also mothers, and I started a lesbian mothers group. We talked about the need for a place where gay mothers could meet each other and explore those two central aspects of their lives. For me it was terribly difficult to blend the two together, to fulfill the responsibilities of motherhood and also to explore my lesbianism. It was incredibly comforting and supporting to realize that there were others with the same concerns.

────────────

When I left my marriage, I recognized that I was moving into something that was dangerous as well as difficult. Being a lesbian could cause me to lose my child. I had "come out" to my husband that morning I gleefully announced to him that I had experienced a lesbian relationship. From then on there was no hiding things from him. He knows what I am, but he has not rejected me as a person or as a parent. If, however, he felt that for any reason my lesbianism was getting in the way of my being a good parent, he would try to get custody of our child. Nothing would stop him from doing that.

Avowed lesbians are allowed to retain custody of their children in about one percent of all their custody cases. A couple of years ago, a woman was allowed to keep her children as long as she did not live with her lover but lived, instead, with her parents; that was regarded by lesbians as a great victory. One of the things that makes mothering as a lesbian so difficult is the constant fear we live in.

It is a major topic in our support group, since many of the members have been through custody cases or are being threatened with custody cases; others are being threatened with loss of their child support or have lost it. I know a lesbian who has not only lost her two young children, but her visitation rights as well.

————

In spite of all the problems and fears, I do not at all regret the path that I have chosen. Last summer, there appeared at my door a beautiful woman who shares many of my beliefs and concerns, particularly those related to raising children. We both feel that parenting is central to our lives and that we want to share the responsibilities of parenting with each other. We want to grow together as parents as well as lovers. We love each other very much — more than I ever dreamed possible — and our love includes love for each other's children.

We knew after we began our relationship that we wanted to attempt to build a life together, but we didn't know how it would work out with her two children and my son. The first time I met her kids, however, they were warm and accepting; it has been that way ever since.

There have been times when the children have tested us and our relationship, and we have wondered how we were going to form this union. We feel very much like pioneers in creating our lesbian family. We parent each other's children and don't feel that the children are exclusively our own. My lover does not feel that I cannot be part of her children's lives, and the same applies with my child. We have attempted to support each other not only in our own relationship, but in our relationship with each other's children.

I prefer to use the word *parenting* because we do not mother in the traditional sense. I'm not taking the mother role, and she is not taking the father role; it is very egalitarian. There is no consistency about which things she does, or which things I do, with the children. I believe that in that sense our children are learning how to live a better way. They see us cooperate; they see us disagreeing; and they see us being loving and concerned with each other. They are learning how to get along without automatic kinds of roles and responses. They are learning more about creatively solving problems.

Because we both have male children, we sometimes have reservations about not having men around for them as role models. However, they each do have their own fathers whom they see and with whom they have maintained relationships. Basically, I think our lesbian family has added rather than detracted from their lives by showing them a positive way of relating to other people, a way of giving and sharing, and a way of being whole. Our relationship is a living example of how two people can join the strengths they have to create a loving environment. And isn't that the best definition of family?

The children are aware that we love each other. They don't know the word *lesbian* yet on a verbal level, and we never call ourselves lesbians because we are afraid that they might use the word with the wrong people and evoke a negative response.

I know that the future will bring difficulties for our children which children of heterosexual couples will never have to encounter. Our kids will have to deal with having parents who are not accepted as being normal. But my hope is that by the time our children are aware of the term *lesbian*, they will have grown strong enough, knowing the love that we have for each other and for them, to withstand ridicule.

NADIA is the pseudonym of a woman in her mid-thirties who has been separated from her husband for two-and-a-half years.

Problems with Sexuality

SANDY BOXER MYLES

From the beginning of our life together, Steve and I had a special, satisfying sexual relationship that gave both of us a lot of comfort and pleasure. It was important to me that nothing change this, not even the birth of our child. As my pregnancy progressed, however, I started worrying that after the baby came, our sex life would be different. If what had happened in my first marriage was any indication, we could say good-bye to sex altogether. Even though I rationalized that my first marriage was wrong from the start, that I was young, unaware, and passive at the time, the fear that the same thing would happen was difficult to shake off.

Talking to friends who were mothers of infants and toddlers didn't do much to reassure me. It seemed as if they were hinting that the months spent caring for a baby were not a time of sexual intimacy for husband and wife. In order to deal with my anxiety, I decided that maintaining a good physical relationship after the birth of a child was a matter of will, and that if this was what I wanted badly enough, I would make it work. I knew the baby was going to create a big change in our marriage, but I was determined not to sacrifice this important part of ourselves.

Without consciously realizing it, I created a Hollywood fantasy of what our first post-baby sexual encounter would be like. After waiting impatiently for the required weeks of abstinence to pass, I imagined we would have a romantic celebration, complete with all the trappings: candle-lit dinner, wine, soft music, filmy negligee, tender phrases, torrid sex, sighing satisfaction. I don't know where I expected the baby to be all this time.

In my rational moments, I reminded myself that it would take some time to get completely back to normal, and that I shouldn't panic or be disappointed if our first attempts were less than perfect for either of us. I vowed to exercise to get my stretched-out vagina and doughy abdomen back in shape so that my body wouldn't be a turn-off to my husband and useless to me.

Things did not turn out as I planned. I was not overcome by a flood of returning passion. The demands of a new baby and nursing around the clock narrowed my desires to one — sleep. Our first sexual contacts were prompted on my part by the lingering need to believe that I still cared about sex and could be true to my game plan. But the "romance" was forced. In reality, I was too exhausted to keep my eyes open, much less get aroused. The baby's sleep habits were totally unpredictable, and when he did fall asleep, I collapsed into bed thinking that, with luck, I could have two hours of uninterrupted rest. When my husband showed up in the bedroom after we put the baby down, I felt ashamed and guilty for not practicing what I preached. All I could think was that sex would cut into my precious time for rest. So I began to calculate coldly how long sex would actually take, and plunged in with one eye on the bedside clock to assure myself that I wasn't squandering more than half an hour. The "let's get this over with" mentality had never been a part of our marriage, and I felt rotten about reducing our lovemaking to that.

I also got caught in a double bind: If I tried to get the whole thing over with as quickly as possible, I was completely unprepared physically and emotionally. My husband seemed like a stranger whom I had hardly spoken to all day, and I was tense and preoccupied with the baby. Under these circumstances, making love was painful and unpleasant. Neither of us got much out of it. On the other hand, reestablishing intimacy and getting aroused took a lot of time, which I felt I couldn't afford; and more often than not, the preliminaries made me feel cozy, relaxed, and very sleepy. Before anything happened, I was out for the count, and my husband's joking comments the next morning had an edge to them.

My exhaustion wasn't the only factor affecting my attitude toward sex. Because I was nursing, I felt that my body was not mine alone. Someone else's life was depending on it. If I didn't get enough rest, my milk supply might suffer. If my husband played with or sucked on my breasts, I thought that I would have to wash them before I could nurse. Since I am prone to getting cystitis, I was afraid certain sex play might cause an infection which would require my taking antibiotics, something I didn't want to do because I was nursing.

I didn't want to take off my nightgown because if I fell asleep naked, I'd freeze and waste time groping around for it when I had to jump up for the baby. As a matter of fact, so many overanxious thoughts about nursing and the baby crowded my mind that I couldn't concentrate what energy I had on enjoying Steve. My body was tensed in anticipation of the baby waking at any moment. I was so attuned to the baby's cry that I imagined I heard him when he was sound asleep. I tried to talk myself into relaxing, but this also kept attention off sex. Steve tried to talk about my obvious lack of response, but I felt ridiculous about telling him some of the things on my mind (he is not a worrier). I concluded with annoyance that he didn't feel the same responsibility to the baby that I did. That and my sense of guilt and frustration translated itself into anger.

In addition to all this, something intangible had happened to my perception of myself. My mental image of "mother" was quite different from that of "sexual woman." I was now a caretaker, a person responsible for another life twenty-four hours a day. I felt neutered. My body had become a functional apparatus designed for nourishing a baby and not for pleasure or enticement. Even though my breasts were big and full — a condition I had spent half my life wishing for — they were as sexless as a cow's udder (and sore and dripping to boot). I slung them around with a total lack of modesty.

I cared little about my appearance. If I was clean and dressed by midmorning, that was a triumph. Since I didn't fit into most of my prepregnancy clothes, I ran around in an assortment of ill-fitting garments stamped with the mark of motherhood — dried spit-up, milk, and urine stains. I looked at my husband as a partner in caring for the baby, but when I saw his naked body, I viewed it with a strange detachment and disinterest. Occasionally, I had enough self-consciousness to think that I must look like a real hot number in my pad-stuffed nursing bra and baggy underpants. I perceived that Steve and I were metamorphosing into a platonic "mommy" and "daddy," shedding our identities of "woman" and "man." Strangely enough, this was happening despite my awareness, preplanning, and desires to the contrary.

I tried to examine why I put myself into a category of female eunuch. Is the selflessness required for mothering an infant incompatible with the "selfness" that is a prerequisite for me to enjoy sex? Couldn't I learn to turn off my weighty sense of responsibility to the baby temporarily? Did I have some kind of neurotic hang-ups about motherhood that dated back to childhood? Was my mother the culprit?

On another level, I was afraid that my lack of responsiveness and appeal would cause Steve eventually to turn elsewhere for sex. That thought got me angry. After all, we were in this together. How dare he look at another woman? What did he think I was supposed to be? I concocted a whole mental dialogue that had no basis in reality. Steve was supportive. He complimented me about my returning figure, and was trying to relate to me as both a wife and a mother — something I had been very vocal about wanting. He was undemanding and encouraging about sex. He bought me a sleek outfit which I secretly regarded as completely inappropriate for me; *mothers* didn't go around in get-ups like that.

Part of me was depressed and angry about the changes in my attitude. Why couldn't we recapture the physical excitement and closeness we once had? Certainly we had sacrificed enough of our lifestyle for the baby. It seemed that if we ever wanted to have some time for intimacy, I'd have to spend a day resting up, trying to schedule the baby (an impossible feat), and getting a brain transplant. So much for spontaneity. And what if, after all this, one of us wasn't in the mood?

As time went on, Steve and I talked more openly about our feelings. He admitted, to my great relief, that since the baby was born, his interest in sex had declined. In the same way I did, he missed the way things had been and sometimes wished we could spend a whole day or evening playing in bed the way we used to, but he was more optimistic about the fact that we would be able to do that again when I stopped nursing and we had some reliable sitters.

I doubt that the answer is just having the time, although that is a large part of it. Something has changed in me. I'm more staid, less spontaneous, more conscious of responsibilities. I comfort myself with thinking that this total immersion in motherhood is a temporary but necessary state of existence that probably has a biological, evolutionary basis, so that mothers will give infants the care needed to keep them alive and perpetuate the race. The most helpful thing to me, however, was a statement made by one of my friends to the effect that after the birth of a baby, a marital relationship will never be the same. The partners will have to find new and different ways of relating physically and emotionally. But this doesn't mean that these new ways can't be as good and satisfying as the old ones. The transition — the letting go of old realities and building new ones — is the hardest time.

SANDY BOXER MYLES has a twelve-year-old son from her first marriage and a seven-month-old infant from her current marriage. In between, she was a single parent for four years. Sandy lives in Metuchen, New Jersey.

11

Ambivalence, Anger, and Shame

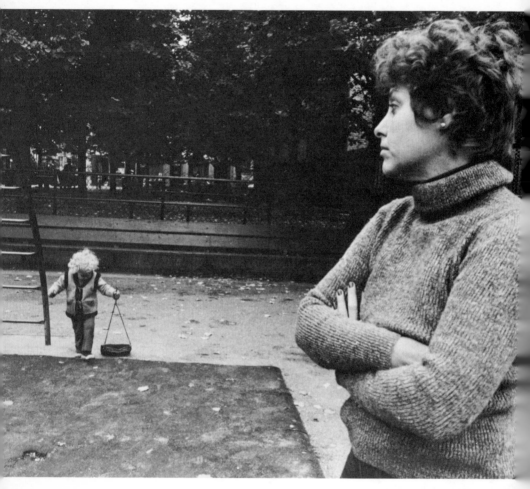

Gail LeBoff

The Children

SUSAN MacDONALD

Sometimes it seems
they came from nowhere,
arrived one Spring,
their quick minds perched on my fence
like precarious birds,
their limbs — wild iris
along my narrow road,

Having erased that time
when love pulled eagerly
at the thighs and the taking of seed
was a contrived joy,
and my belly, a ripe, golden sun.

It is as if
I never planned to bear them
turned suddenly to a gift
   of young voices.

Yes, they are here, and firm
eating my days — wind rascals,
ogres.

I love them,
wanting them gone.

Both Sides Now:
Ambivalence and Motherhood

SUSAN LEWIS COOPER

Seth is two and a half. I adore him with a passion I never imagined possible. To me, he is bright, beautiful, and charming. He can also be demanding, insistent, stubborn, and loathsome, and during those times my fantasies include child abuse. This is an essay about ambivalence; it is also about an ongoing internal struggle.

A colleague of mine once remarked that the "terrible twos" are a child's way of helping the parents separate from him or her. I understand that concept completely. I am surely less reluctant to leave Seth when he is having a tantrum on the floor than when he is happily engaged in an activity. Although I realize that mothers have both positive and negative feelings toward their children beginning from their birth, I was only mildly aware of my negative feelings toward Seth for approximately the first twenty months of his life.

Sometime, shortly before he turned two, I became aware of how much Seth understood about my personality and emotional character. He knows my maternal strengths and weaknesses; he knows where I am vulnerable; and he knows which of his behaviors hurt and anger me the most. He has also learned strategies that tend to distance my husband and me from each other. He knows, for example, that as much as I try not to show my feelings, when he announces that "I like Daddy better than you," if I'm feeling particularly inadequate or insecure at that moment, a rash of negative feelings gets triggered off in me, from anger to hurt to jealousy. I might then be tempted to offer him a treat in an effort to "win him back." If, however, I am feeling reasonably good about myself, and secure in my role as a mother, I know that he probably likes his father better at that particular moment because I have denied him something he wants.

I also realize that when at other times he strongly prefers me, it is still his way of getting what he wants. In my more secure moments I let myself be sensitively aware that at this point in his life he too is feeling many ambivalent emotions. If I am feeling confident about my mothering, I can hear his announcement as a statement of preference in a given moment, and not as an overall indictment of me as a mother. I can then respond to him reasonably, allowing his preference to stand, without giving in to his demands. Even when I am feeling basically good about myself, however, and Seth's ability to hurt me is severely diminished, some hurt and anger still manage to seep inside. It is testimony to his power.

Since my responses to Seth are often a reflection of how I feel about myself at a particular moment, I worry about the effect that my inconsistent responses may have on him. My worst fear is that he will become emotionally disturbed. And although I know intellectually that there is no basis at all for this concern, emotionally the fear remains, sometimes barely perceptible, at other times blatantly present. I think about the shameful irony of being a practitioner of mental health whose own child is disturbed.

I have discovered that parenthood is filled with intellectual dilemmas that are often more difficult than the ones I solved in graduate school. The most mundane issues often prove the most challenging. What do I do, for example, when Seth, who has just asked me for juice, has a mild tantrum when I hand it to him in his blue cup? When he insists repeatedly, "I want it in my Oscar the Grouch cup," do I quickly pour it into the cup he wants, thereby both avoiding the unpleasant scene and encouraging him in his search for autonomy and self-determination? Or do I state emphatically that his juice is already poured, that he doesn't have to drink it, but that I am not going to dirty another cup? Does being firm and refusing to be manipulated by a child ensure that he will not develop into a demanding, spoiled adult who constantly insists on having his own way? I ask myself these questions practically every day. Although I have no answers, I usually comfort myself with the belief that even asking the questions helps me in my struggle to be a good mother. Perhaps it is my search for answers that keeps me going. Sometimes I love all the challenges of motherhood; sometimes I would trade them all for a fifteen-minute massage.

Whether I ultimately choose to pour the juice into a different cup or refuse to do so, the point is that I often feel like dumping it over my son's head. If his whining and insisting go on for a long period of time, my thoughts about what to do become more drastic. I occasionally fantasize about hurting him physically, although my distress about child abuse has become more intense since I have become a mother. I have two strong, though seemingly contradictory responses to that deplorable phenomenon. I cannot even read stories or articles about child abuse; it pains me so to think that innocent children can be tortured by their own parents. On the other hand, I understand emotionally how it happens, since in my worst moments with Seth I have fantasies about hurting him physically. Fortunately I know that I have enough control over my impulses not to act on them. But I no longer put child abusers into a separate category — "us" and "them." Perhaps it is because most of my physical, material, and emotional needs are satisfied that I am able to exercise restraint when necessary. If my basic needs were constantly being frustrated, I doubt that I would be so in control.

———————

Somewhere deep inside me I believe that a good mother is soft-spoken and calm at all times, even in the midst of children's crises and tantrums. She is unquestionably loving and tender in her behavior, and never allows angry feelings to show. She is always willing to play with her children, or to give them attention when they ask for it. In short, a good mother's feelings, wants, and needs are subordinated to those of her children. As I write these words I feel ashamed. Intellectually I no longer believe them. Powerful feminists have convinced me otherwise, and I too have attempted to convince other women that they have rights — as mothers, workers, wives — that include meeting their own needs. For some reason, however, these relatively new beliefs do not apply to me; emotionally I am living in an earlier century.

I feel an inexplicable pull inside. My love for my son is profound; I know it is unconditional. I want to be a good mother, yet I hear myself yelling at him often and feeling frantic at times. I have witnessed myself yanking Seth's arm to get him moving, even in enjoyable moments with him. I often say no to his requests to play with me. In fact, I would probably be rich now if I had a dollar for every time I've said, "I'm too busy right now." And I feel guilty when I opt to stay in bed in the morning while announcing to Seth that "Captain Kangaroo" is on television. Emotionally I have "rules" about good mothering. Behaviorally those rules often do not apply. The truth is that although I am deeply connected to and in love with my son, my feelings about him and about motherhood are mixed, confusing, and continually changing.

In thinking about ambivalence, I am reminded of Newton's third law of motion: for every action there is an equal but opposite reaction. I think that the first law of mother-emotion is that "to every feeling there is an equal but opposite feeling." I recall the times I have left Seth at his day-care provider's house, with tears in my eyes, longing to be with him, and cursing my job that was keeping me away from him. And yet there have been many other days when I questioned whether I could remain sane until it was time to bring him to day care. I am aware of the joy I feel when Seth greets me after a day at family day care with open arms and a huge grin on his face. And I am also aware of the guilt and hurt I feel when he ignores me or says, "I don't want to go home now." When he says, "I love you, my mommy," my chest fills with love. When he ignores a question I have asked him several times, or a request I have made, I get furious and the love turns to hate.

For the first few months after Seth was born, I tiptoed into his room each evening before going to sleep to make sure he was still breathing. My attachment to him was so strong that I feared he would die and that I would fall apart. Now, not because I am afraid that he is going to die, but because I enjoy the ritual, I tiptoe into his room each night, cover him with his quilt, and kiss him lightly on the forehead. Sometimes my husband joins me, and we both gaze at our son. At those times, I know only that I adore him and that I would never, never — even if I had the power to do so — wish that he did not exist. Although he is a separate human being, I am connected to him in an incredibly powerful way. It is frightening and it is thrilling. And although I know that the following day will include all the polarities of emotions I have previously described, each night, in those moments before bedtime, I experience no ambivalence.

SUSAN LEWIS COOPER, in addition to being a mother, managed to finish her doctoral program course work, write her dissertation, work part-time as a psychotherapist, teach a few courses, and co-author a book.

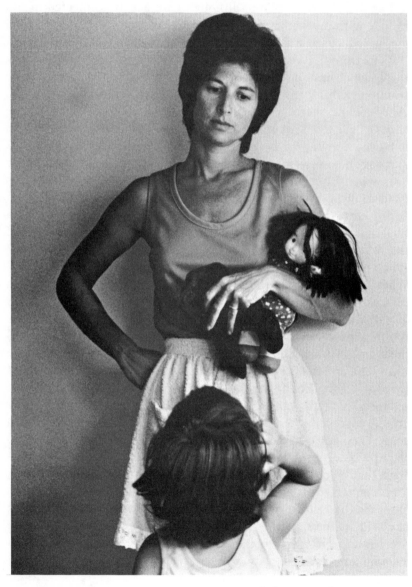

Ethel Diamond

Preferring One Child

DOTTIE CRITCHLOW

Is it possible for a conscientious mother to prefer one child over her others? Until the birth of my third child I would have said an emphatic no, but as I was to learn, situations change.

Micki and Danny are my children from my first marriage. I remarried two years ago. Shortly thereafter, my new husband lovingly and legally adopted my children as his own. One of our goals was to strive for a normal family life that would nurture each of us.

After the initial adjustment period, we decided that we were ready to have a baby. Sara Beth was born nine months later, and I was ecstatic. I was the mother of three with love to spare.

Once home from the hospital, full-time mothering responsibilities quickly depleted the reserves of energy and love that I had earlier experienced. Because my time and energy were limited, Sarah Beth's needs received top priority. Micki and Danny had to wait for what I had left. I didn't feel that I loved them any less than before, but I did notice that I felt drawn to Sarah Beth and guilty about how much I enjoyed caring for her. Micki's and Danny's interruptions, even for basic needs, irritated me. Before long, I was comparing my other two children to Sarah Beth. The new baby represented the joy and fulfillment that my life had been empty of in my first marriage. Micki and Danny sometimes reminded me of my past and of the most miserable times of my life. It was easy to see some of Lee's features in Sarah Beth, and it was hard to ignore Micki's and Danny's physical resemblance to their biological father. Lee's intense interest in Sarah Beth was something that I had never experienced with my first husband when his children were born. Also, nursing Sarah Beth created an emotional-hormonal bond that I had not enjoyed with my bottle-fed babies.

Micki and Danny seemed to need even more attention than before the baby's birth, and I resented their additional demands on me. It sometimes felt like an obligation to care for the boys; I felt drained by them. Often I found myself wishing that my past had never happened, so that there would be just Lee, Sarah Beth, and me.

When I finally shared my feelings with Lee, he reminded me that I could not change my past; I could not change who Micki and Danny were, or who they looked like; and I could not deny my special feelings for Sarah Beth. Somehow, I had to gain control of the emotions and fatigue which were stifling my ability to be the mother I wanted to be to *each* of my children. I knew that I did want to love Micki and Danny unconditionally. I decided that I needed to learn to appreciate each of them as individuals again. Looking at their baby pictures helped me remember that they also had been special infants to me. And it helped Lee to see what they had been like as babies and toddlers.

I realized that a contributing problem was the fact that the boys were now older, school-age children who were becoming independent of me. I didn't know how to handle their new growth patterns and behavior stages. Once I began to read books on child development, which taught me what to expect, I became as excited over the older children's progress as I did about the baby's daily accomplishments.

It would be nice if I could say that I no longer favor Sarah Beth, but some days I do; then I experience the same feelings of guilt. I've learned, however, to handle these feelings more constructively. I make an extra effort to be involved with my other children, and I spend time with each of them individually. I've slowly learned that difficult situations can change.

DOTTIE CRITCHLOW was twenty-seven when her youngest child was born. She is a "happy, stay-at-home [Grove City, Pennsylvania] mother."

The Abused Child as Mother

ELIZABETH MOODY ALLEN

Several months ago I celebrated my thirty-fifth birthday. I was feeling a little neglected, depressed, and abandoned. I had not received a single card or phone call from any of my three sisters, brother, father, or friends. Being alone with my two children was a reminder that I am estranged from most of my family. The central explanation for this lack of contact lies in the rippling effect of the physical and emotional abuse my sisters, brother, and I suffered as children from our parents, and in particular from our mother.

I have spent much of my adulthood measuring myself against a vow made in my adolescence never to be like my mother. Though I have never beaten — as opposed to spanking or slapping — my children, I have felt great rage toward them. I have felt uncomfortable with this anger and have feared that one day I might not be able to control the fury.

As an adult I have expended much energy hiding the truth of my battered childhood as if it were a disease for which I would be labeled hopelessly deviant and unlovable. The shame I feel for my parents' behavior has somehow been absorbed, but I am constantly hoping that it "doesn't show." Despite my intellectual understanding that it was my parents' problem, and that I am a "successful" adult, a secret, small part of me feels indelibly wounded — not crippled, but scarred in some terrible, unseen way.

My children, a son sixteen and a daughter ten, were quietly doing their homework. My heart was pounding as I asked them if I had ever told them about some of the things that happened to me as a child. (Of course, I knew I had not.) They both looked up.

I began by describing the "who-done-it" game my mother would repeatedly use in order to elicit an admission of guilt by one of us for a misdeed. She demanded that the guilty one "own up," otherwise we would all "get a lickin'." She claimed that she could tell who was lying by looking into our eyes. No one would answer.

The tension would mount as the seconds passed. The spanking began with me, the "privileged" number one. Her favorite implements were hairbrushes, yardsticks, and, on one occasion, an asphalt shingle. All beatings were administered on bare flesh. I told my children how I would volunteer to go first. That way, at least I could get it over with. I would hear the others crying and screaming in the background, waiting for their turn.

I told my children how I took great pride in never crying. My sixteen-year-old son's eyes widened as he commented, "Ohhhh, and I bet it made them hit you more." I replied that it did have that effect. My decision not to cry was an attempt to maintain some control and not to let her break me. At least I retained my self-respect.

My heart stopped pounding. I felt a warm current of acceptance flowing from my children. They said things like, "Gee, that must have been terrible." I was relieved that they were not upset or denying the validity of my experience. I hoped that if at times they thought they had a terrible mother, my childhood experience would give them some perspective. I felt encouraged to go on.

One evening when I was about ten, my mother started the who-is-the-guilty-one routine. Someone had gotten toothpaste on a washcloth. No one would admit to the "crime." She filled the bathtub. One by one, she called each of us over, ordered us to lean over the edge of the bathtub while she pushed our heads under the water. My ten-year-old daughter interjected loudly, "I wouldn't go. What did you do? I would have run away." My son said quietly, "No you wouldn't." My children's words were a gift to me — a gift of understanding.

My son sat up on the couch, and my daughter put her books aside. I went on. When I was fourteen, my mother suddenly stormed into the room I shared with one sister. She screamed that she hated me almost as much as she had when I was twelve. She turned on her heels and stormed out. I was astonished. Turning to my sister, I had laughed and said, "Gee, what did I do? I didn't know I was so bad now or when I was twelve. What did I do *then*?" Obviously her hatred for me was irrational and not based on anything I had "done."

One Sunday afternoon, when I was sixteen, my sister and I had gone, with permission, to the local teenage hangout. My mother called after we had been there about an hour and shrieked into the telephone that my sister and I should "get our asses home." No amount of pleading or questioning why she had changed her mind altered the demand. As my sister and I walked the mile home, I rehearsed a venomous speech. My anger was rising to boiling. My sister pleaded with me to calm down, to please not do it. A whole childhood of controlled anger welled up within me into a blind rage. I stormed through the house straight up to my parents' bedroom, where my mother spent much time in front of the television set. All I remember saying — screaming — was that she wasn't the mother around here. She was nothing but the warden. Suddenly I found myself sprawled on the floor at the top of the stairs. My father had silently bounded up the stairs behind me and with a single blow had knocked me down. He continued to kick, stomp on, and yell at me. Time and feeling were suspended. He finished by picking me up like a rag doll and tossing me through my half-open bedroom door. My head struck the door as the rest of my body slammed into a bureau. I was instructed not to come out of my room. I silently got into bed and pulled the covers over my head. (My sister later told me in horror how my mother had sat in bed silently watching the scene with a smile on her face.)

I did not tell my children the sequel to this violence. No one came into my room for a long time. I felt numb. I had not even cried. I just wanted to go to sleep forever. I quietly got out of bed, went to the bathroom, and sneaked a bottle of aspirin back to my bed. I started swallowing the aspirins dry. I had taken only about ten pills when my sister came into the room, saw what I was doing, grabbed the bottle, and threw it to the floor. Aspirin scattered and rolled everywhere. I felt totally defeated. I couldn't even kill myself properly.

I had worried that telling my children about my parents would be upsetting, especially since my son has shown great interest in family history. Then I wondered why I was protecting this Sunday-portrait image of my mother, who has been dead thirteen years, and my father, who has never remembered my children's birthdays nor been to my house in over a decade. Part of me wants to protect family members whom I care for very much. There is another part — a very angry one — that would like to see the truth cut deeply into my parents' histories. All the understanding in the world for my parents' immaturity and problems will neither give me back my childhood nor erase the pain of my mother's frequent, snarling remark, "If it weren't for you kids . . ." How could I apologize for being born?

The ensuing discussion with my children was one I will never forget. I was attempting to put the extensive violence of my childhood and the relatively little violence I have directed toward my children into perspective. Even for this small amount I feel guilty. I hoped that my children could now better understand why I have made such a issue of nonviolence, especially in the past few years.

Yes, my children had noticed that I had not hit, slapped, or squeezed their flesh for over two years, since I had resolved that I would never strike them again.

My daughter, however, recalled the times when she was little when I would squeeze her face in "controlled" anger. She demonstrated on my face. What a déjà vu feeling that was! I told her how sorry I felt now — and then — that I had hurt her. "Boy," she said, "I sure didn't like you very much then!" I gathered myself together and replied that I could understand because I sure didn't like my mother either when she hurt me. I asked her if she remembered how she used to come downstairs from her room after a fight and sit near me with her "blankie" over her head. She had looked like a little ghost. My heart would go out to her, and I would gather her up into my arms. We would rock together and promise to be "nice girls."

My daughter looked at me sheepishly. She must have sensed that I had needed her forgiveness as much as she had needed mine. This was something I had never received from my own mother, who neither acknowledged the violence nor apologized for punishing those who were not guilty.

I have been frightened that I have always had more intense feelings for my daughter than for my son. Her misbehavior triggered my anger much more easily than my son's. It seemed as if I was trying so hard to be the good mother to her that my own mother wasn't to me that her misbehavior highlighted my failure to be the perfect mother.

My son's even temperament, in contrast, has caused me to joke about how I thought I was a "good" mother until my daughter came along. I have not known how to evaluate these feelings. It reminds me of the farcical statement my mother often made that she loved all of us the same. I didn't know about the love part, but I was certain that she hated us differently.

———

I have experienced another violent relationship — with my former husband and the father of my children. He and I had been in psychotherapy for six years in order to save what I have only recently acknowledged was a violent marriage. The violence had been denied for several reasons. Because I had never seen my parents strike one another, and because I had erroneously thought that only adults who were criminal hit each other, I was absolutely shocked when he first hit me. I was then eighteen years old, married less than a week, three months pregnant, rejected by my parents ("I had made my bed . . ."), and in college a thousand miles from "home." I felt trapped and deviant. I had no more control over my life than when I was a child. His violence and mental torture were little more than an extension of my mother's.

My husband's violence took place in front of the children only once. It had been several years since he had last hit me. After his recovery from a near-fatal series of operations, we were left physically, emotionally, and financially drained. I had made many personal sacrifices to keep the family solvent. The recurrence of the unpredictable violence was a most excruciating betrayal. After a long struggle, we had finally become successful, affluent, professional members of a small community, and he felt confident that his violence toward me would have no repercussions. He remarked, "Who would believe you?"

My decision to leave him was directly tied to the violence. I reasoned that staying in a violent marriage would teach my children that violence is acceptable behavior. It would also be saying that I didn't value myself, or my life.

When I secretly made plans to leave, I found neither my family nor my friends would take me and my children in; they feared violence for themselves and their families as retribution for helping us. My attorney's advice was to protect myself, since the courts are notorious for their ineffectiveness in restraining violent husbands. One can only guess the power of the messages my children have learned about the real vulnerability of women.

When I discussed with my therapist my intention to leave, I

was advised not to go, but to try a little longer to work things out. But I chose life over emotional — and possibly physical — death.

The violence of my childhood and marriage has been a deep, dark secret which I have hidden from most of the world. My mother served as a negative model, someone whom I didn't want to be anything like. As a mother myself, I have been plagued with mental acrobatics. Am I really like my mother after all? Is the rage which other mothers have reported sometimes feeling toward their children really like what I have felt? I have tried to overcompensate for my lack of being parented by loving my children as I would like to have been loved. And I have tried to make up for their father's lack of parenting.

With time, I have finally come to realize that I cannot make up for the deficiencies in my childhood and that my children's experiences are entirely different and separate. I cannot relive my childhood in an improved form through my children, but perhaps I can learn to relax now that I know I am not like my mother, and that I do not have to repeat her mistakes.

ELIZABETH MOODY ALLEN is the pseudonym of a woman attending college in New England.

My Daughter, My Rival

REBECCA M. THOMAS

My transition from wife to wife-and-mother was complicated by feelings of jealousy toward my new daughter, in addition to the normal uncertainties of first-time mothers.

Because I needed to recuperate from an emergency Caesarean delivery, my husband took over the majority of the child-care tasks.

I was amazed at his seemingly natural skill and adeptness. He, not I, was the first to show our infant off to visitors. Although he had been nonchalant throughout my pregnancy, he radiated with pride over his new daughter.

I had wished for a spontaneous delivery, and I was feeling very inadequate and a little less than a woman because I had not had one. I also felt useless because I was doing so little around the house and helping so little with our baby. Watching my husband spend a great deal of time with our daughter, I began to feel jealous of her. While I held and nursed Mikala, I was overcome with love and tenderness. But when she took up my husband's time, I began to fear that she would also take my place in his life. Subconsciously I wanted the love she received to come only from me.

When I finally found enough courage to share my guilt and feelings of jealousy with my husband, things improved dramatically. He had not even realized that I had been harboring such feelings; he had attributed my irritability and rejection of him to normal postpartum depression. Once aware of the problem, he made a conscious effort to divide his time equally between the two women in his life. My feelings of jealousy quickly dissipated and were replaced by shame that I had ever felt that way.

REBECCA M. THOMAS became a mother when she turned twenty. She was born and raised in Jacksonville, Alabama, where she lives today.

From Super Child to Problem Child

CAROLE GREGORY

Jim was an incredibly bright baby. He walked early, started talking at seven months, and spoke in whole sentences at fifteen months.

How amazed we were when he sang the alphabet song and counted to twenty before he was a year and a half. He met every developmental task without difficulty, from giving up his bottle at a year to toilet-training at twenty-six months. He was also marvelously sociable with adults — a very affectionate and extroverted child.

I felt blessed, happy, and proud. I spent a lot of time reading books to Jim, singing songs, playing games, and talking. I was eager to be with him. "After all," I would say, "this is my work: motherhood is my job." When he did something precocious, I glowed. I accepted his misbehaviors, such as smearing Desitin all over his room, and responded with a stern but good-natured reproof. No chore was too taxing; all was done willingly. Merely watching Jim grow was rewarding.

That is why I was not prepared for what happened. When Jim was three and a half, my world caved in. A wild, uncontrollable child greeted me when I arrived home from the hospital with his brother, Mark. I hoped that once we got back into a normal routine and I had time to be with Jim, I could allay his fears and he would calm down. But he didn't. He became more frantic and difficult.

───────────

During my second pregnancy, I had wondered how a new baby would fit into our lives. My relationship with Jim was so close and precious that I questioned whether I would resent the baby as an intruder. Ironically, Mark was so dear and trouble-free that he became my refuge from an increasingly hostile Jim. I could cuddle and love Mark while Jim was at school. When Jim was home, I had to spend most of my time with him so as not to arouse further jealousy. I hoped to reassure Jim, but he did not respond to my efforts. He would constantly handle his baby brother roughly, and David and I were unable to stop this behavior with discussions, warnings, or even punishments. Also, Jim became increasingly physical with his playmates. I had to monitor his play because he would strike out aggressively or have a tantrum when he was frustrated. I felt angered and drained whenever I witnessed one of these scenes.

I had always believed in "reasoning" with Jim. He was so intelligent that I expected him to control his behavior once he understood that his actions were improper. Suddenly, the basis of my approach to mothering was no longer viable. I was losing my ability to control myself. My anger was exploding into frequent episodes of yelling, followed by exhortations of why Jim should want to behave. Even we, his parents, the proponents of rational behavior, were being provoked into hitting our child.

I was further shaken by his nursery school teacher's report. Jim was her most difficult behavior problem, and she recommended that we seek professional help.

How could such a thing happen to my bright, wonderful son? How could Jim, my source of joy, have changed so radically, and over such a short period of time?

While Jim's difficulties may have been triggered or exacerbated by starting nursery school and the arrival of a new brother, I realize now that certain characteristics were present in his personality before they later became so readily apparent. Jim viewed himself as a miniature adult; he was therefore committed to having his own way. As the only child of two adoring parents, he experienced few clashes of wills. But when our family included a new member, and when he was asked to fit in with a group in school, his willfulness and inflexibility caused him serious problems.

I can now offer this rational explanation for his behavior, but at the time I was profoundly confused. I felt betrayed by my child; how could he do this to me when I had given him so much? I was embarrassed by the way he was acting and sure that everyone was wondering what kind of mother I could be to have raised such an uncontrollable "brat." Jim and I had been so close. I saw raising him as my job; and he was therefore my product. He was an extension of me and proof of my worth. People actually stopped seeking us out, thus reinforcing my sense of rejection and isolation. The play group I had organized when Jim was eighteen months old started meeting in secret without us. When one play-group mother met me in the nursery school parking lot, she tactlessly told me: "The women in the play group used to talk about Jim, how active and difficult he was. Tell me, what did you do wrong in raising him?"

Admitting that I needed help was easy: I was desperate to change the situation. David was supportive, but he was rarely home, so the burden fell on me. We never blamed each other for what had happened; but we knew that we didn't have the answers. Before

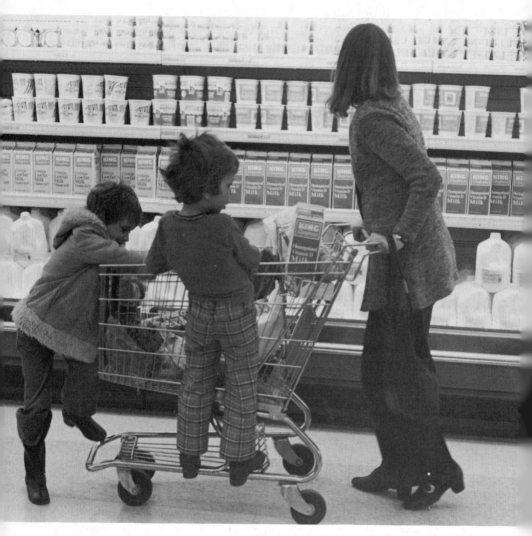

Joan Albert

Jim's birth I had been a counselor, and I was well aware that the right person could help us effect the necessary changes in our lives.

We spent six weeks with a social worker who seemed eager to point an accusing finger at us, an approach which annoyed David and added to my guilt and depression.

Next we ventured to a psychiatrist who tested Jim for brain damage, gave him tranquilizers, put him on a special diet for hyperactive kids, and finally administered Ritalin. None of this helped. And I suffered additional remorse over giving Jim drugs.

Mercifully, the search ended when we met a perceptive, competent psychologist. The first time I met her, I sat there and cried, "Jim's ruining my life." She immediately understood and offered concrete suggestions for improving the situation.

She emphasized that she believed that I had been a good mother. She helped me to stop feeling so guilty and being so defensive.

I learned that I was the boss, not my three-year-old child. Jim was relieved to know that there were firm limits and that I had set them. He fought against my control, but we both knew that I had the power to enforce my rules. For example, formerly if Jim hit someone, I would say: "Hitting is against the rules and now we must go home." He would scream and kick and force me to drag him down the block. I would feel impotent, embarrassed, and angry. Now I would add: "If you come home quietly and cooperatively, you will only have to stay in your room for fifteen minutes and then you can go out and play again. Otherwise you will be in your room till dinner."

It worked. When Jim knew the rules and the consequences, he would control himself, reinforcing his belief that he could control himself. My confidence was strengthened, and I felt like an effective mother again.

I also stopped explaining everything ten different ways and sometimes answered his "why" with a simple "because I said so." I no longer intellectualize with Jim; to him, that is a word game of explanations, excuses, and denials. He must cooperate because the situation necessitates cooperation. I no longer run a democratic household: I have become autocratic.

I have learned not to feel that I am being judged by Jim's behavior. He is not an extension of me. I try to stay out of his play and his school, sparing myself the aggravation and allowing him to deal with the consequences of his actions. If he is unpleasant with other children, he will be rejected. If his behavior at school is not appropriate, his teachers are trained to handle him.

The situation is not perfect, but at least I am now less ego-involved. If I'm angry, it's because he's getting on my nerves and not because I feel personally betrayed. Occasionally I slip back into old patterns. At my first parent-teacher conference this year, I still felt as if I were going to get *my* report card, not Jim's. It is my nature to be impatient with my own imperfections, and if I slip back into thinking of Jim as my extension, I become impatient with his imperfections as well.

I continue to work to accept my child as he really is, not an idealized version but an actual person with strengths and weaknesses. I take delight at Jim's positive accomplishments and attributes, but I am more wary and my joy is more reserved. I still become angry with Jim, and I'm not always a model of controlled behavior. But I also believe that my being less than perfect will not harm my child. I am working to accept myself too.

CAROLE GREGORY is a pseudonym.

12

The Only Child

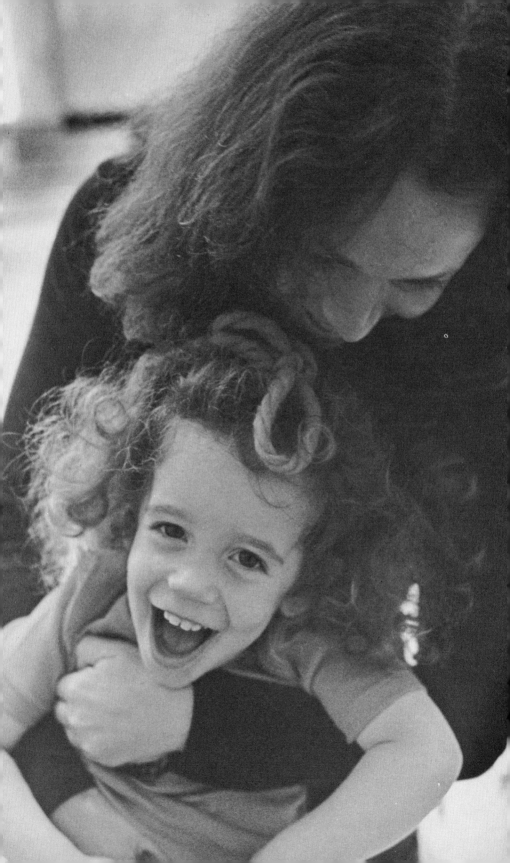

One Is Enough

NANCY PAROLINE HOOK

My two-and-a-half-year-old son is an only child and he always will
be. Mothering him has enabled me to see and feel much without
which my life would have seemed empty, but I am not ready to
make a career of washing diapers and stumbling from bed to bed at
three in the morning.

My husband and I moved to central New York over three years
ago, he to start work as an engineer after graduate school in North
Carolina, and I to begin some sort of career. Our feelings then about
children ever being in our lives were more negative than positive.
First and foremost, we decided that we could not afford a child.

But within two months, I was pregnant. My husband blamed
me for the pregnancy. He was worried about our finances and feared
that by having a baby at that time we would ruin all later chances
for a happy life. I was frightened of the future too, and resented the
child for the rift it had created between my husband and me. But
I had made the decision to keep the baby — for moral reasons I
could not have had an abortion.

Even at that time I was fairly sure that this was to be my only
pregnancy. I really hadn't wanted any children, and the physical
discomforts I later endured — nine months of backaches and bleeding, ending with twelve hours of hard labor — only reinforced my
feelings.

Clearly I did not initially want a baby, but my son is loved
more than words can express. It is important to me to perform as
best I can as a mother. I worry constantly that the decisions I make
may have terrible repercussions in Ben's adult life. Contrary to the
common belief that, with each addition to the family, child rearing
becomes more relaxed, I know I would care deeply about each
child's development. Being responsible for Ben alone leaves me no
freedom to respond to my own needs. I don't wish to complicate
matters further by enlarging our family, and Jerry agrees.

My relationship with Benjamin is so intense that we often exclude his father. I fear that another child would affect my relationships with both Ben and my husband. And I fear that I wouldn't have enough time and energy to give adequately to a new child.

Mothers of two or more children have told me that when they came home from the hospital with a helpless, tiny infant, it was difficult for them to find love for a cantankerous, demanding older child. In my own family of eleven children, the second youngest, who had been the baby for four years, became an unruly brat when the youngest was born. It was hard for us to analyze her feelings of displacement; it was easier simply to cut her off from our affections, which only served to fire her resentment more. I do not think it would be fair to put Benjamin in such a situation.

Since Ben was one year old, friends and relatives have been asking when we plan to have another baby. They advised us to get it over with so that the children would be out of diapers at about the same time. But how wrong it is to cut short a child's babyhood, a time when he truly needs his parents, merely to eliminate washing diapers or other similar inconveniences.

Those well-meaning urgers of large families smile knowingly when I protest that one child is enough for Jerry and me. They are certain that when Ben gets older I will want a little one to fill my arms. That may be true, but I will also be relieved that there is no longer a little one filling up all of my free time.

Ben is just now old enough to help rather than to hinder, but still much of the day is spent dressing, bathing, feeding, and picking up after him. It will be a long wait until the spontaneity of the pre-Benjamin days of our marriage returns. Merely to be able to go outside without the worry that the baby is drinking poison or breaking the china would be a welcome restoration of some of my freedom.

————

We have also been warned that Ben will become spoiled and lonely if we stop our family at one child. We see it differently. To us, Ben is the lucky recipient of our special attention. From Ben's birth, my husband and I have tried to be his best friends. We give him our time and energy, instead of substituting toys or other objects, as many busy parents must do. Because my day is not exclusively spent in the laundry room or in front of the changing table with two or more babies, Ben and I can read a book, go outside to pick wildflowers, or just sit around and play with our dog. I am always nearby to explain that monsters are not real, laugh when he pretends to be nursing a football, and show him a chickadee at the bird feeder.

We realize that Ben needs children of his own age to play with to prevent him from becoming a know-it-all "adult child." Although our neighbors' children are much older or younger than our son, and although we live in a fairly isolated area, we have found ways to accustom Ben to playing and disagreeing with children his own age. Once a week, for example, he attends a play group with three other boys. His temperament and ability to share have already improved in the few months that he has been in the group. I also exchange baby-sitting time with other mothers, to give Ben a temporary playmate while I run errands. Much as I enjoy caring for the other children, I must admit feeling relieved when the doorbell rings and their mothers return. The baby sitting is a small taste of what it would be like to have another child, and it makes me realize how deeply I cherish my short times of peace and quiet.

Perhaps we are depriving Ben of certain joys and experiences inherent in having brothers and sisters. Certainly, my own siblings are close to each other. We all know, even if we would not have chosen each other had we the option, that we will always be there for each other when needed. In spite of this, I would not want to be pressured into doing what others assume is right for our child or for us, and then resent that decision for the remainder of my life.

Should I accidentally become pregnant again, I'm sure that the initial despair would give way to resignation and hope for a happy future. Underlying the motherly exterior, however, resentment and feelings of imprisonment would always be ready to surface. I don't know whether any child would be able to handle those feelings, no matter how seldom they were expressed, or if it would be fair to live with them. For us, one is enough.

NANCY PAROLINE HOOK grows and presses flowers, which she arranges and sells at local fairs and shops. She lives in Cazenovia, New York.

On Being and Having an Only Child

MARION FISHMAN

I was an only child — I gather for much the same reasons that my son Daniel is. My mother had several miscarriages after my birth, and she finally gave up trying to have more children. I never even conceived again, for reasons as mysterious as my taking three years to conceive and then, for no particular reason, doing so. Our guess is that between planning to adopt and busily stripping and painting the walls of nine rooms in our first house, the pressure was off and the psychic cork popped.

I grew up in the country, a mile from the center of a very small town. Being an only child in an isolated area was a very lonely experience, in spite of my parents' efforts to get me together with my friends. As their marriage deteriorated into frosty, quiet antagonism, I wandered the woods behind our house and poured my heart out to my cat. None of my peers shared this experience; we did not grow up in an atmosphere where discussing personal feelings was encouraged. Although at the time I was probably not so aware of it, I later believed that having a brother or sister to talk to and share the horrors of separation and divorce with was something that I would have given *anything* to have had.

I told myself that I would never, *ever* have an only child. I would not want to expose my child either to the intensity of feelings and expectations unbuffered by siblings, or to the loneliness I had felt.

———

My husband Paul's feelings were similar, although they underwent an interesting development. He was functionally an only child because his younger sister was born retarded and placed in an institution when Paul was young. Before his parents made this painful decision, Paul suffered her destructive rages, and afterward he endured the guilt of knowing that she was sent away — in part — so that he could flourish. Because of this, he, even more than I, became the object of his parents' expectations, hopes, guilt, and overprotectiveness, plus their complicated reactions to giving up one child for another. He too wanted his son to have a more normal atmosphere in which to grow.

As Daniel grew and I aged, and we began to anticipate my getting pregnant again, Paul's fears that a second child might be retarded, as his sister had been, grew also. What we discovered, after the initial disappointment of my not getting pregnant again (in spite of many tests and thermometers), was that having one child was really "okay." Given our pasts, it felt familiar. We had a good sense of what daily life would be like for our only child, and for ourselves.

I also found that my desire to begin motherhood again waned as I returned to part-time social work and became not just a wife and mother, but wife, mother, *and* professional. Furthermore, our thinking about having been only children evolved to the point where we believed that Daniel did not have to suffer the disadvantages incurred by us. Paul and I are fairly adventurous types and do not have serious inclinations to overprotect Daniel. (In fact, a friend of mine jokingly labeled me an "underprotective mother.") We know also — as far as one can know — that we will not inflict divorce upon him. We are aware that it is important for him to have easy access to other children if he is to learn to give and take. And we try to restrain ourselves from making him the object of too many expectations.

There are some things, however, that you can't make better. I will never learn not to listen for every "pearl" of wisdom that falls from his lips. Only the fear of a future daughter-in-law hating me keeps me from treating Daniel like a prince (and some realization that he could become a spoiled brat if I am not careful). I also wonder if the fact that Daniel is spared the insults and insensitivities that siblings sometimes hurl at one another is positive or negative. Is he better off for the delay in being told that he can be "boring" or "dumb"? Of course he will have to cope with those issues with his peers; but will it become more difficult for him because he did not have to deal with the harsh realities earlier in life?

The most painful aspect of having an only child I have saved for last, because I can hardly bring myself to think about it, let alone write about it: the vulnerability. If something terrible should happen to our child, who is everything to us, could we survive?

Would having other children protect us from an unbearable loss? I will never know the answer to this question, but it haunts me.

Daniel now thinks that being an only child is terrific. When he is older, he may regret lacking that special tie which only siblings share. We have made a concerted effort to live in neighborhoods with many children his age. And, like my parents did with me, we invariably include one of his best friends in our outings and trips. We hope he is learning about negotiating with people through very close contact with his peers; I wish I had had more of that opportunity.

There are definite disadvantages to our two generations of only children: not only does Daniel have no siblings, but there are also no aunts, uncles, or cousins. To compensate, we have developed an "extended" family of close friends who have become "aunts" and "uncles" to Daniel. These relationships have become tremendously important to all of us, and we take them very seriously.

Growing older is a constant process of facing realities and giving up illusions. It never occurred to Paul and me that we would re-create so closely our own family constellations, or that our experiences as children would have such an effect on our parenting.

MARION FISHMAN gave birth to her son "after what seemed an endless battle with infertility." She currently works half-time as a social worker and also maintains a private practice out of her home.

Considering a Second One

CAROL KORT

My daughter is now two, and I am thirty-four. It is time to think about having a second child. Much of me wants to have more family: I love it when other children are around Eleza, when she is involved with her peers instead of clinging to my leg; I love the idea of siblings and family gatherings, the chatter and cacophony of family feuds and emotional resolutions. For me, blood ties are the bottom line in life. Yet I am uncertain, unresolved.

———————

I am the conflicted one. I ask myself questions: Do I have the capacity to restructure my life all over again, as I did after my first child was born? Will I have the patience I had for one child when there are two? I am used to Eleza, and she to me. Will I resent an intruder into the lovely relationship I have established with my daughter? My husband does not ask these questions. He feels ready to have another child; he misses having an infant around the house, and he is certain that we will manage, somehow, at every level. I am the conflicted one.

I have my body back. It took me so long, postpartum, to feel sexy and attractive again. I become angry when I think of all the stretching and ballooning my body would go through if we had another child, and then all the months it would take for recovery. Being older could only make it more difficult physically.

I have my work back. After months of guilt and struggle, I feel perfectly comfortable with my arrangement of working part time and having Eleza spend her mornings in a family day-care home, close to where my job is. I know that I will want to work soon after a second child is born, but I become frightened when I think about having to deal with two day-care situations: the car pooling, the adjustments, the harried life of a mad housewife dropping off this kid and then that one, arriving at work exhausted before beginning the day.

I have my life back. I have limited but precious periods of free time. When Eleza is napping, or with her father or a baby sitter, I can be with friends and have a normal uninterrupted conversation; or I can be alone. I become panicked when I think about having to care for the infant while the toddler naps, and vice versa; or about spending my "free time" with my older child so that she will feel as loved as she felt before the sibling arrived. If we have another child, would I ever find time for *me*?

I see a newborn on the street, and my heart melts. I desperately want to hold her. I miss the milky sweetness of nursing, the softness of a newborn's tummy, the vulnerability of a clinging infant.

─────────

A close friend calls to tell me that she is pregnant. Her first child and my own are about the same age. I am thrilled for her and feel a rush of envy. But then I feel relief that it is not I. The thought of a second child immediately evokes excitement, desire, doubt, and fear, in no particular order.

I look at my maternity clothes, and I feel ill. They are dumpy and depressing. My daughter is napping while I'm doing this, and I am grateful to have some time alone. I push the box of clothes aside and decide to have my diaphragm refitted. I love our compact unit of three. I want nothing and no one to change it.

I have dinner at a friend's house and am warmed by the caring of a family of six as they clean up together, giggle and mime silly stories, and give and take from each other's experiences. I wish Eleza had aunts and uncles who lived nearby. I wish she had more than one first cousin. Our little world of three appears tame and withdrawn compared to the interaction of that larger family. We are missing something.

─────────

I know too much now about what can go wrong. It is uncanny how many birth defects and tragedies deluged close friends soon after I had given birth to Eleza. Suddenly a dear friend had an infant who inexplicably lived for only seven hours; another gave birth to a dwarf — spontaneous mutation. I am distraught at what could go wrong with a second child. After all, if I was lucky enough to have a child without real problems, why should fate deal me another perfect hand?

I watch my daughter with a playmate. I observe that she is generous, that she is not aggressive enough, that she takes turns and makes jokes. When her playmate leaves, there is a heavy silence in the room. I can sense Eleza's very real need for siblings. I decide that I want to become pregnant immediately. I want more family. I want another baby.

─────────

I remember making the decision to have Eleza. My husband and I had married young and had therefore grown up together, quite literally. We did not like to depend on anyone else, or have anyone depend on us. We were free spirits who lived spontaneously and on very little money, moving from one decision or experience to another without too much planning or concern. Having children did not fit into our unhampered lifestyle. And I never particularly liked children or felt liked by them. I lived in an academic community where everyone was charming, bright, and childless. At one point, on the spur of the moment, we decided to spend a year in Israel. This decision — the ultimate expression of our childless way of life — was, ironically, the pivotal event that changed that way of life forever. Living on a kibbutz altered my attitude about family and children radically. The entire orientation of kibbutz life is on family, cooperative living, and having children. It was the antithesis of the quiet, adult, self-centered world to which I had grown accustomed. I began, slowly, to feel comfortable around children and families, and with the maternal feelings burgeoning in me. When we returned to this country, we had Eleza. It was the best decision we have ever made.

But there is no kibbutz to help me out with my current dilemma. I realize, too, that there will be no epiphany to make this decision conclusively for me. When I think that Eleza would not be if I had decided to forgo having children altogether, I want a tribe. When I think about that realistically, I am sucked into the total exhaustion of one child, let alone two, and I am once more back to the heart of the matter.

Holidays are cheerless without children to celebrate them; even with one child, our plans are too easily made, too easily broken. Chaos is natural. I hate the perfect order of my home when Eleza is not around. There is lifelessness in things being clean, still, and unaltered. I begin to wax philosophical and see the necessity of a large family as a natural, disruptive, and humane force.

Motherhood has unquestionably been a peak experience in my life. Getting there is another story. Even given my easy pregnancy and delivery, I do not look forward to having to go through either stage again. Who needs all that perking and brewing when it is far less painful to order the instant brand — especially the second time around? Yet I am too egotistical to consider adoption unless I have no choice. I want more of my own flesh and blood.

I am the conflicted one. I want the luxury of more time to worry about whether or not to have another child. But as I approach thirty-five, I do not have indefinite tomorrows for childbearing. Spiritually, and to some extent emotionally, I am ripe and ready. The poet Rilke says that ripeness is all. But am I overripe, becoming a shriveled piece of fruit on a vine that has given up its best fruit already, and now wishes to be left alone to grow leaves instead of being laden with fruit? I attempt to listen to my intuitive voices, but still I cannot hear the answer.

This is the period when questions are raised. If we have another child, I will forget these questions and be too in love, too involved, and too busy with the infant to remember that they were ever asked. If we decide not to have another child, I will forget the answers and concentrate only on the questions. I will rationalize in order to feel comfortable with my decision.

On one side are intangibles: love, family, nurturing, the universe. The other side encompasses real, everyday tasks of a mother who is stretched to her limits and is wary of adding anything or anyone else to her life. But that same mother has always found room for more love, energy, and time when she deemed them necessary. She is pulled by large forces, and by small ones.

In between the questions and the answers lies another life, or not another life. Will it somehow be decided for me, and not by me? No, it is a difficult decision but such a meaningful one that I must accept the responsibility for it.

I fold the drab maternity pants with the frayed elastic stretch waistband and place them back in the box. Then I put the box away — for now.

13

---

*Becoming
a Single Mother*

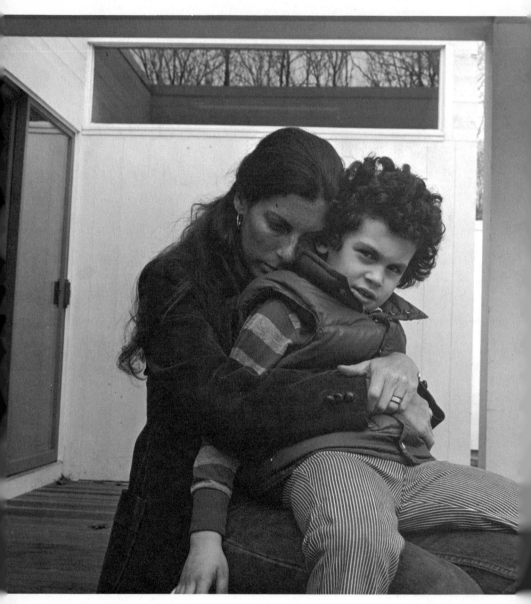

Birgit Blyth

On Our Own

JACQUELINE STRESAU

The birth was wonderful: brief, powerful, exhilarating. Between summits of pain, I watched my son come forth into the bright air of his new world, and had no idea that I would raise him alone.

The early months at home with this tiny being who spent most of the day asleep, breaking his dreams only long enough to fill his belly, gave me many long hours for reflection. By the time Brenny was four months old I was aware of a pervasive staleness in my four-year-old marriage. Worse, I saw that I had married Tom largely out of deep-seated fears about being alone in the post-college, adult world. My need to be taken care of had blinded me to the reality that I had little in common with the person I married.

It was many more months before I could sort all this out and come to any conclusion about the marriage. Brenny flourished in spite of my turmoil. My favorite time with him was early evening, when I would cradle him in my arms and softly sing him folk songs as the day slowly shifted into night.

After an unsuccessful attempt at marriage counseling during the fall Brenny turned two, I decided to leave the marriage and to keep Brenny with me. At the same time, I terminated individual therapy, finally feeling free of confusion and eager to begin a new life.

I moved from our little house in suburbia to a new neighborhood closer to the city and to good commuter bus lines. I thought that when Brenny had adjusted to the changes, I would find a part-time job. In the meantime, Tom was providing enough financial support for us to manage.

The first month was marvelous, my mood as sparkly as the Christmas lights that swooped across the streets. I felt free to pursue interests that I couldn't share with my husband — psychology, sensitivity groups, the new literature on psychic phenomena. I could spend time with anybody I wanted, for as long as I chose. And there were no more tiring hours at the ironing board, steam-pressing Tom's business suits.

On Christmas Eve, Brenny and I flew on a tiny, six-passenger plane to a warm holiday with my big, fun-loving family. Brenny, the only little one in the clan, was the star of the celebration. I relaxed and delighted in all the attention my terrific child was receiving.

It was not until the flight home that the other feelings surfaced.

As we approached the city where my real life awaited me, my stomach twisted and tightened. I looked out at the blue and white quilt of sky and thought, I am alone. No one is down there waiting for me: no husband, no parents, no sister or best friend. There is no one to look out for us but me.

───────────

At morning coffee klatches we met the neighbors, women who kissed their husbands off to work and took care of their houses and their small children each day. They talked of school programs, sales, new babies on the way — of lives going on as they always had. I sat mute and alienated, but Brenny enjoyed playing with the children, so we continued going.

Icy, white January. I was sitting at the kitchen table watching Brenny dribble cereal when forgotten incidents began streaming across my mind: little lies, careless oversights, unthinking remarks, mean comments to my brother. From childhood to the present, I recalled twenty-eight years' worth of things I wished I had done differently. For weeks, I couldn't turn off the barrage more than a few minutes at a time.

Late at night the thoughts shifted toward the future. What was going to happen to me in my old age? Would there be poverty, cold-water flats? I pictured Brenny's childhood and adolescence; I couldn't see him growing up happily.

Brenny's wake-up noises always came too early. Dull and aching from the night, I only wanted rest. But there was no one else to care for Brenny. Resolutely I hauled myself out of bed each day, changed the soaked diaper, began breakfast.

Monday, Tuesday, Wednesday . . . each day was alike. Mornings I did housework while Brenny played with his toys. If I sat down to read or talk on the phone, he would clamber on my lap and jabber to me; so I saved these activities for his nap time. In the pale light of late afternoon, we either walked to a bookstore to browse or picked up groceries. Suppertime was lonely. I invited friends over when I felt up to it.

On the days that I was very tired and Brenny squirmed a great deal while I changed him, I yelled and slapped. He cried; sometimes I cried along with him. These incidents provided still more material for the tape of wrongdoings that ran on in my mind.

By late February I found that I could not concentrate on long conversations, television shows, or books — unless they dealt with depression. Taking walks in the damp remains of winter only increased my sense of dreariness. I knew that I had never felt like this before; my teenage bouts of depression had always been brief and temporary.

Brenny began to ignore his toys and stare out the front window, sucking his thumb. I picked him up, held him, patted his butterball body. But inside I felt like dried-up cardboard.

Spurred by friends, I tried to find a job. But at interviews I felt wooden, thick, unable to focus. There were no offers. Luckily I was still able to make it on child-support payments.

Therapy had helped me in the past, so I went to a nearby clinic where I was assigned to a very nice social worker for weekly visits. One day I blurted to her, "I just want someone to take care of me." She decided I needed a full-fledged psychiatrist.

I felt washed out, wilted, lethargic. At one point I asked my therapist if he thought hospitalization would help me. His enthusiastic response shocked me. I hadn't been serious. Entering a psych ward would mean losing custody of Brenny. And, above all, I was not going to lose this child. Part of my determination came from a core of love for this small being who needed me for his own survival. And, too, on some obscure level, I knew that Brenny kept me — if tenuously — held together, reminding me that I was me, the same woman who had given birth to him with pride and strength two-and-a-half years earlier.

On Saturdays Tom picked up Brenny for the day, and I rushed out to buy new toys, seeing right through my own eagerness. In the long afternoon hours I lay on the living room couch, unable to think of anything to do. Inevitably my thoughts went to the bottle of sleeping pills in the medicine cabinet. I pictured walking into the bathroom, pouring out all the red capsules, and gulping each smooth little cylinder. Then I jumped ahead to the part where Tom would return, holding Brenny's small, round form in the deepening twilight, neither of them knowing why I didn't answer the door. I couldn't go on with the fantasy. That scene, I knew, would never take place.

I saw my lawyer for a rehearsal of the divorce hearing. When he asked me why I felt I should be awarded child custody, I fumbled over my words, hesitated, and came to a dead stop. My attorney pressed me; I started to cry. He asked the name of my psychiatrist, saying that he needed final word from my doctor before calling off the hearing. Reason: plaintiff not fit.

In therapy that same day, I could do nothing but sob.

"Is there anything you've wanted to do in life, besides raising a child?" The doctor's words were very soft.

Another burst of tears. I had been a good student in college, fascinated by literature, writing, and the study of other cultures. But none of these things could compare with the sweet, dark-eyed child who had once lived in my own body. Taking care of Brenny was the only thing I was attempting to do, and I couldn't even seem to do that.

Once I was alone in the car, deep animal moans welled from my chest. I drove slowly through damp April streets, watching the procession of gray buildings, wet sidewalks, reaching dark fingers of trees.

My mother drove across the state to help out for a week. Although I knew it would be difficult for her to see me in this kind of shape, I couldn't pull myself together. I had never been able to put on cheerful faces when feeling unhappy, even in the best of times.

Together she and I agonized over the options. Should I attempt the hearing? Should I — unthinkable to either of us — simply give up child custody? (Shared custody was not among our choices; the practice was almost unheard of in the small midwestern city where I lived.) What about going back to Tom? For the first time I considered it, now that I'd seen how hard it was to cope alone. Wasn't there a chance we could live together peaceably, contentedly, even if without rapture? Perhaps my sights had been set too high.

I called Tom to talk it over. We went out a few times, enjoyed simple dinners, and talked about Brenny, Tom's new job offer, the future. I felt better with him than I did when I was alone. Eventually my husband agreed to try a reconciliation, mostly — I surmised — for the sake of his son. I was banking on the hope that once inside my little family, I would feel like myself again.

Immediately we flew to the East Coast, where Tom's new employer was located. I basked in the security of marriage and in the long-awaited summer sun. Feelings of strength and warmth returned, flooded high, and spilled over to Brenny. In very little time, his disposition turned as sunny as the weather.

Although I felt as good as ever, and less dependent on Tom than in our earlier relationship, one major problem remained: our marriage had no life in it, no depth of understanding. When I got involved in a writing project and forgot to vacuum the apartment, Tom lashed out, "I think you need psychiatric help again. You just don't seem to be happy being a wife and mother like everyone else."

He was right: I wanted to be more than a wife and mother. I was happier when I spent time writing. Tom didn't want to visit a counselor who could possibly help us cope with our difference in outlook; I saw no way love could develop without a base of understanding.

Again I opted for life as a single mother. Feeling strong and optimistic, I made plans to travel back to the city I had left a half-year earlier. I didn't really think about how Brenny would react to the move; I was too caught up in my own preparations.

I arrived with no place to live, no job, no car. Friends helped me find all three, however, and this time I chose an apartment near a couple I knew well. Three-year-old Brenny entered nursery school, while I began part-time work as an administrative aide. Though my chief qualification was high school typing skills, the job was worth a great deal to me: money of my own; a sense of connection to other adults; and the feeling that I was contributing to the world outside myself.

Often I was tired; usually I was broke. I still lost patience, especially when scrambling to get Brenny and me ready on weekday

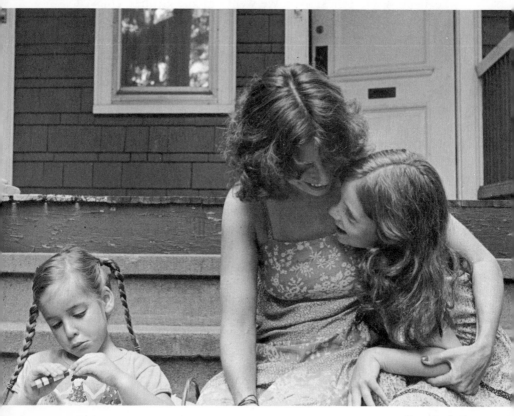

Bonnie S. Burt

mornings. And as the brisk winds of winter blew against my window panes, I again began to feel closed in and isolated.

But something was different this time. My heaviness was not so weighty, my inner aching not so persistent. Now I had a feel for who I was and what I could do — separate from Tom and my family. But I also had to deal with Brenny's changes. I found out about his method of coping with a life halfway across the country from his father when his baby sitter asked to talk to me.

"I didn't know whether to tell you about this," she began tentatively, "but finally I decided I should. Every time I come here, Brenny goes through this 'thing' — a time when he won't play, won't eat, gets real sad, and talks about his father. About how great everything was when they were together, how his father took him everywhere, carried him piggyback, spent every day with him, always laughed and told jokes. He'll go on like this, talking and crying for a half-hour or so — and he won't let me change the subject. Then, all of a sudden, he'll stop. As if it never happened, he'll start playing, eating, whatever he was doing before — all smiles."

At fourteen, she wasn't sure what to do about these episodes. I told her that the way she was handling them seemed terrific, and gave her some details of the separation. She seemed relieved and eager to keep helping.

Once she was gone, I sank into a chair and wept. Three years old and initiating therapy, following an instinctive urge to do exactly what he needed to do. I was moved by Brenny's trust in his baby sitter, and amazed at his ability to express himself.

Painfully I realized that Brenny was feeling very sad and that he wasn't ready to talk about it to me, his mother. I felt bad about this, but I understood: because of frustrating issues surrounding the divorce proceedings, I had been feeling very angry with Tom. Although I was careful not to express this hostility in front of Brenny, he picked it up with the special "radar" children possess. I resolved to become more open to Brenny's thoughts and feelings about the split.

We were lazing around on a Sunday morning when I had my chance. The subject of the break-up arose; I began explaining the reasons in a simple, matter-of-fact manner. Brenny stopped pushing his truck on the sofa, looked straight into my face, and told me emphatically, "An' it's sad."

I saw his brown eyes glisten; I noticed the tremble lurking about his chin; I heard his absolutely clear statement.

There was nothing to do but to agree with him. Happy as I was to be finally on my own, there was no getting around the fact that for Brenny the break was sad. My task was to empathize without feeling guilty about leaving Tom — a difficult undertaking. Although I wholeheartedly believed that one reasonably happy parent was better for a child than two discontented parents, all it took was a flash awareness of Brenny's pain to bring a torrent of guilt rushing through me. Why had I been so blind about the marriage before I had given birth? Why hadn't I recognized clues that must have been there from the beginning?

There were no answers. I had to learn not to ask myself tormenting questions, to lift my thoughts from the finished past and set them firmly in the present — the everyday events going on around me. I learned that when I let myself get too low, my warm feelings for Brenny began to dry up. And I discovered that I could maintain my vitality by establishing caring friendships with other adults.

In time Brenny's pain subsided. Emerging from a quiet shyness, he began to enjoy romping with friends at school. During the second summer after I left my husband, he stayed with his father while I visited my sister in Boston. Brenny thoroughly enjoyed his time with his daddy, and I liked Boston so much that I decided to stay there, returning to the Midwest only to pack and to retrieve my son.

————————

Boston was so enticing — with its plethora of adult courses, hiking groups, coffee houses for lingering — that staying home with Brenny sometimes felt like a jail sentence. I angrily envied the childless freedom of my sister and of my work colleagues and friends. At the same time, I loved coming home from the sedate work world of adults and falling into a tickle tussle with a five-year-old bundle of giggles. I constantly walked a thin, unclear line, balancing my own needs against those of my son. There were no road maps, no formulas, no models for this way of living.

Joining a women's support group — a warm, safe place to bring feelings — I discovered that other women felt lonely; other mothers felt trapped, resentful, and impatient some of the time. We talked; we listened; we felt our way into each other's lives.

I took up meditation and found that it gave me a kind of command over my mind's wanderings, helping me reduce negative thoughts. In meditation, I could step aside from my problems and gain fresh perspective. And I could contact a deep, enduring part of me that was not shaken by day-to-day events.

When Brenny took his first flight alone to visit Tom that summer, I went out to celebrate two weeks of single, carefree life. In fact, I went out every night of the week, to make up for lost time. Freedom! I could do whatever I wanted, whenever I wanted: stay in town after work, hear an evening poetry reading, stay out until two in the morning without worrying about baby-sitter costs.

And something else happened during those two weeks. Early in my "vacation," one lunch hour, I wandered through the park to a playground. Children were all over the place — scooting over monkey bars, madly swinging, laughing, shrieking. I sank to the grass, my eyes fastening on a chubby boy of five or six. My arms ached to swoop him off the ground in a giant, gushy hug.

Each day I returned and sat by the playground, gazing, absorbing, feeling my eyes grow moist. What was I doing here? I could be lunching with a friend. I could be shopping for new sandals, or taking in a noon concert. But here I sat, watching a bunch of kids run wild over a patch of green in the middle of Boston, my ears throbbing in the loud, marvelous clamor.

The whole time I was childless and free I could not stay away from the playground. I was a woman, a growing self, a wild-flying spirit. And — through some mixture of circumstance and crazy, wonderful luck — I was also a mother.

JACQUELINE STRESAU is the pseudonym of a writer of promotional material, poetry, and humor.

An Unmarried Mother

SUSAN ELLMAN

I vividly recall discussions my mother and I used to have about how difficult it was for her as a mother to do what she believed was right, despite social pressures and our pleadings. Looking back at those talks, I see that implied was the assumption that I would, of course, become a mother. But also implied was the thread of conviction that I always carried with me: motherhood required careful thought and decision making. I always considered mothering to be serious work.

When I met my future husband in college, our earliest games involved what we would name our children, even though during the four years of our marriage I had no desire to have children. I had gone through a serious illness and in some sense had reverted back to childhood feelings of tremendous vulnerability. As a feminist, I viewed my friends as downtrodden and oppressed by the weight of motherhood, whereas I valued my own independence and freedom. I recognized all the ways in which I had betrayed my true self as a child in order to get approval, especially from my parents. A rush of anger overwhelmed me, particularly toward my parents, and generally toward society at large, for what they and it had done to me and to all children. I witnessed adults using various methods to force children to conform to society. I certainly did not want to join the ranks of the oppressors. In addition, I was gripped by the horror of the Vietnam War and the idea of bringing a child into this world seemed, at best, meaningless.

Fortunately, I did not remain in the clutches of this negative world view for too long. With the rise of the women's liberation movement, and the end of the Vietnam War, things changed. There was a real sense of hope and opening up of closed doors. In my own personal life, the change resulted in an attempt at an "open marriage" (for lack of a better phrase) in which my husband and I wanted to retain our commitment to each other, while allowing each other greater freedom. To this day it is bitterly disappointing to me that we did not achieve this goal; and I still believe that it is not an impossible one.

216

During that period of allowing other relationships to enter into our marriage, I met Michael, a man with whom I could share my positive political and spiritual feelings, who also was willing to share the mundane and tedious aspects of everyday life: laundry, cooking, bills.

After a trip together across the country, I returned thinking I was pregnant. The onslaught of positive feelings surprised me. Suddenly I remembered those talks with my mother, and I knew I could love a child. Many issues and questions, however, complicated the picture and clouded those good feelings. Could I support a child economically? Would I resent the demands a child makes? Would I have to give up my new-found sexual freedom and my less-than-conventional lifestyle? And would I want to be responsible twenty-four hours a day for another human being? The old ambivalence returned, but the context for having a child had changed drastically. The circumstances — the father of my child would not be my husband — were far different from any I had expected.

As it turned out, I was not pregnant after all. But a new attitude and interest in children had emerged. I began to watch and relate to my friends' children and to see what beautiful and complex beings they were. At the same time, I ran into a woman I knew from the women's movement who was pregnant and looking for someone special to watch her older son and forthcoming infant while she returned to teaching. It presented the perfect opportunity for me to discover answers to some of my questions about mothering without taking the plunge itself. For the next two-and-a-half years, I grew and learned and loved with these two children. I was privy to a whole new world of children and the people involved with them. Besides the valuable information I gained about myself and how I relate to children, I was able to develop some criteria for the environment in which I could consider raising a child. That environment would have to be one in which the child had more than two adults with whom to bond, and where the adults had more freedom and space than could be found in the nuclear family.

My interest in collective living had developed gradually. But I was very fearful of what I imagined would be a sexual free-for-all, and a situation in which I would have no right to privacy. I was also afraid that I could never adapt my living habits to those of the others in the group, and that my needs for neatness and order would be put down as "bourgeois" habits. Later, as I listened to the women in my two consciousness-raising groups discussing the breaking-up of their marriages and how finances were becoming tighter and tighter, many of those fears were replaced by anger at how difficult it is to "make it" in our society. It is often overwhelming for two people to have full responsibility for children, home, and jobs; but for one, it can be crushing. While many view collective living as risky and requiring great courage, I now see it as more secure and less anxiety producing than the traditional family unit. As more of us remain or become single, our needs for a community increase. The holidays that used to call for strictly family get-togethers in the past have become gatherings that now include extended family — friends and roommates.

───────────

My own collective living situation has expanded to include five adults. Through a series of incredible events, one of these five is a childhood love over whom I had suffered when I was sixteen. Despite the fifteen years of separation, we found that what we had felt then had been quite real, and adulthood has only enhanced our ability to share and communicate. While his return to my life was a source of tremendous joy to me, it created a very painful and difficult struggle with Michael, with whom I had been living for about four years. Although we had always agreed that there was room for other people in our lives, the reality put us to the test. Our determination, and the willingness of our newest household member, helped us work and fight to stay together. We did not let sexual insecurities or guilt prevent either of us from continuing to share the life we had built together. We prevailed over the very same internal and external pressures that had partially been the cause of the failure of my marriage.

About a year later, I became pregnant. That childhood crush, back in my life as a lover and housemate, was to become the father of my child.

Once it was real, and not merely intellectual conjecture, all the conflicts and decisions with which I had grappled had to be reexamined. My criteria for collective living were met; I was living with people who were caring and loving. I also knew that I had the love and interest needed for this undertaking. And I was delighted that my child's father was someone whom I had so long cared for, and who was so essential in my life. He was legally separated from his wife and had two children for whom he was responsible, whom he loved and felt tortured over having left. Many issues had to be considered: Could he handle another child? Could we handle having a child outside of marriage? Was it right to take that on in terms of ourselves and our families?

I had spent years after my divorce trying to rebuild the relationships with my family and my in-laws. And now I was about to explode everything again. The possibility of my parents' rejection was also very real, and the thought that my child might lose the special relationship with them as grandparents was painful. I was also worried about the reactions of the baby's other grandparents. What it all came down to was this: if it were not for the rest of the world, I would have been thrilled. I felt that, like my mother, I could not let the rest of the world determine my decision about what was right. I had to listen to and trust my own feelings and those of my baby's father. And so we proceeded.

Much to my surprise, once the initial shock wore off, my parents were not only accepting but very supportive. The relief and joy over that acceptance contributed greatly to my enjoyment of my pregnancy. In addition, my friends and sisters in the movement provided encouragement. Strangely enough, all those "downtrodden mothers" were happy and pleased for me. One issue, however, did become a source of concern, especially to my parents. They believed that the baby should have its father's name; I wanted it to have mine. The name I had chosen to retain was my married name, because I felt that the person I had become was identified by that name. Unless I chose a completely new name, any family name would have been a man's name. It became clear to me how strong the tradition of patriarchy really is. Our baby would have the same name as only one of its parents, yet it was assumed that the one would be the father's. Because the father had already had the experience of children carrying his name, I felt I had a right to the same experience. While we feel as committed to each other as we both know how, we also are aware that life offers no guarantees. And if I should some day be raising our child without him, I would want the baby and me to have the same name. The father respected my feelings, and though he was not in complete agreement with them, we arrived at a compromise that satisfied us both: we gave the baby his family name as a middle name.

We both agreed that marriage, even if it were possible, was not something we wanted and needed for ourselves. If at some future time this becomes a source of difficulty for our child, we will have to reconsider this decision. I thought a great deal about how many women have gone childless because they never found the "right" man to marry them, and how many women have endured miserable marriages because what they really longed for was children. Progress has been made in allowing single people to adopt children, but the stigma still exists over a single woman bearing her own child.

In addition to these other questions and complications was the factor of Michael's role with the baby. Initially I had wanted both men to be present during the labor and childbirth. But I became overwhelmed by the number of obstacles involved in accomplishing this when dealing with a hospital birth. I decided that I could not face that struggle at a time when I would surely feel vulnerable and in need of reassurance and support from all quarters. It was very difficult for Michael, a friend and former lover, not to feel left out during the pregnancy, despite his sharing one-third the cost of the delivery. I counted on the baby to capture his heart and resolve that pain once she arrived, and in no way was I disappointed. After much thought about what to title the relationship between Michael and Sara, we decided on "godfather," because it is one that society can recognize. Also, in Michael's Greek culture it is a significant and important title. Despite many tensions involved in collective living, one area of tremendous joy to all of us has been relating to Sara. Both men have also taken great pleasure in witnessing my happiness with her.

───────────

Because I was ready at this time in my life to share myself with a child, I have not resented the demands. Because I live collectively, the burden is not mine alone. It was impossible for me to have known or understood ahead of time the rewards of relating to my child, despite my experiences with other children. Recently there has been much written and said in the women's liberation movement about the oppression that goes along with motherhood, and much of that is real. But more women are also beginning to allow their positive feelings about mothering to emerge. Instead of giving up motherhood itself, they are struggling to change the conditions of mothering. To me, *that* is the crucial goal, and certainly not to do away with it altogether.

SUSAN ELLMAN lives communally in Long Island, New York, with the father of her child and four other adults, including her sister. She was one of the founders of the Women's Liberation Center in Nassau County, New York.

Absentee Mother

BARBARA N. BIDDLE

The bulky yellow school bus heaves into sight. I kiss my two younger children, Peter and Eleanor, and they climb aboard. Through the fog-streaked window I see their faces as if I were looking at an old, out-of-focus slide. The bus backs up ponderously. We wave good-bye. In the afternoon, I will be gone. On that day and every school day thereafter, they will be met by their father, Bill. We talked to them about it and explained it. It was like preparing children for surgery, but no one asked, "Will it hurt?" The two older boys, Bob and Ed, comprehended the news in their own ways. Ed, at sixteen, simply said, "So what's new?" But Peter, eleven, crying with us on a walk down to the river, told us that divorce was the worst thing he could imagine. No one asked, "Why?"

Recently Bill told me that if he could do it over he would fight harder to keep me. We acted civilized but were actually terrified of our own and each other's anger. We played our roles magnificently; however, neither of us knew where they would lead.

What does it mean to walk out of a family with a couple of duffle bags, a tennis racquet, and a typewriter? I felt as if I were going to summer camp. I alternated between knowing for certain that leaving was justified and right, and believing that I was insane. Emotionally I was unable to deal with the power of what I was feeling; so I went numb.

I know that ideally children should be raised by two loving parents. Nonetheless, I had to leave the confining, possessive love of a man whom I first met when I was fourteen and married when I was eighteen, after one semester of college. Being married was hard for me. Our life together was in a constant state of tension caused by his desire to enclose me and my attempt to pull away. He dreaded abandonment and I suffocation. We were hopelessly, neurotically interdependent in ways that stifled both of us.

During my relationship with Bill, I became pregnant five times and gave birth via Caesarean section to three sons. We adopted our daughter.

I kept order in a house that resembled a dormitory. For ten days each spring, Bill made maple syrup on the kitchen stove in huge kettles. In winter, he greased his boots in the living room. Scores of mountain-climbing expeditions were planned and outfitted in our front room. Crampons, ice axes, tents, packs, and pots were stored in our entryway. My sons followed their father's example by bringing their ten-speed bikes into the house. We owned thousands of books, magazines, and catalogs. Bill's students were in and out at all hours. When I cooked it was simple, wholesome, and in large quantities.

When the boarding school where we lived rented space one summer to National Training Labs, I took a giant step and joined a ten-day Human Growth Lab as a scholarship participant. I finally stepped out of the relationship as a separate person, and my marriage was unsteady from then on. I expanded my activities to include attending college part time, writing, yoga, and consciousness-raising, always searching to add more meaning to my life.

Still, our family was the most important reality for me; without children, I doubt that my marriage would have survived five years. There were moments when I would be so warmed and cheered just by the sight and sound of the children that I knew I would never be as happy again. But I also knew that our children would grow up and leave home. And without them, there was not going to be enough to sustain me. To wait would make it even more difficult for me to join the work force and become self-sufficient, and I needed that terribly.

Our decision that I would leave Bill with the younger children was based on the fact that we could not afford two households. The boarding school where we lived provided us with a house and most meals in the dining hall, which is a huge supplement to a private school teacher's salary. At first I planned to make a "home" for the two younger children when I got established, but child-support payments would have left Bill without money for toothpaste. I couldn't stay and kick him out of school housing; besides, I didn't want to live in that community anymore. I also realized that the children would have been torn from the security of a small-town school and the love and support of our fellow faculty members and families. My leaving them there seemed like a sound and rational solution.

Bill wanted to keep the children, there was no doubt of that. He has extraordinary energy. He is basically a good and kind man and has the advantage of knowing what he wants and almost always getting his needs met. The children live where he works, and if one of them is sick he can hold classes in our living room. All maintenance is taken care of by the school, and once a week a hard-working cleaning woman comes in to shovel out the place. Bill is a good single parent, but I doubt that he or any woman friend of his can replace me as a mother.

I loved being a mother. Without that comfortable and familiar role, there is a nagging ache of "something" missing, like the pain of a phantom limb. I remember all the fun I had with my children — the jokes and teasing, the playfulness and the wrestling matches. I also remember a ten-week siege with chicken pox, as one child after another came down with it.

I miss being needed. There is no longer a toddler hanging on to my leg or a lanky teenager handing me the car keys. My new housemates are not too receptive to hearing my views on sex, God, death, and morality, which I used to share freely with my children.

Each time the children visit, I am more convinced that I am losing the intimacy we shared. I know that mothering has to be continuous with young children, that it means being present when they need you. They can't save up their needs for three weeks until they see me again. I no longer know what they are thinking, doing, learning, suffering, or what they want. Even if I were to see them more often, it would still be strained. We are missing too much of each other's lives. The parent who does the caretaking gets the goodies. And there is much about my life that I can no longer share with them.

I sometimes wish that I had a spyglass trained on the house. The news I get is often upsetting. Apparently Peter does not read my letters. My old rocking chair, the one I rocked Peter and Ellie in when they were infants, is broken. I guess what I want to hear is that it isn't the same without me, that they miss me, but that it is okay.

I get some satisfaction knowing my children can manage without me, that they have gained enormous independence. They choose their own clothes, get ready for school, decide what to do with their free time, know when they are sick or tired, pack their duffles to visit me, and cope without the things they forgot. I hope that they are drawing on some of the strength I left behind.

Now when I see my children, I reach out and they vanish like little ghosts. We spend entertaining and educational days in Chinatown, exploring, or roller-skating. But I feel like their aunt. I try to encourage them to talk about their feelings, yet I am as afraid of opening up as they are — I might cry. When I tried to share some of my deeper feelings with Ellie, she just nodded and didn't respond. I cannot play therapist with my own children. They need their defenses. Although they know that I love them, I led them to believe that I would always be there. They expected to grow up and leave *me*. If a mother can change like that, they must be frightened that anything might happen.

I can only guess what my children's feelings were when I left. We met at the Aquarium, three weeks later, and all maintained stiff upper lips. Peter says now that at the time he was extremely unhappy. Yet I know that he and Ellie were glad to be in their own beds, not in strange ones. I suspect that Ed felt angry to be left with his father, but the best choice was for him to stay with his schooling. Bob probably felt that he had already lived through it once: two years earlier I had made an abortive attempt to leave during the year he was studying in England. I'm sure he suffered greatly being away from home at that time.

I can't deal with their unexpressed feelings; I have my own private hell of guilt, grief, fear, and lost love. In their own time, I hope that they will talk freely to me and that they will be able to forgive me.

What sort of person does this make me? I am a puzzle to some, an anathema to others. What I have done is scandalous, unpopular, and threatening. I had spent most of my life trying to please people, so this is risky business. But I'm struggling to find my own genuine and authentic self, and not everyone can approve of the path I've chosen to take.

Why did I give up the myth of a happy marriage? So far my new life is very meager in affirmation, satisfaction, and fun, but I've just begun. I am angry that we didn't have enough money so that I could leave like a conventional wife and set up a household with children, ample support, furniture, and a car. I feel enormous sadness and loss, and some regret. I am lonely and alone often, and having my children would lessen that pain and give me a role that I know well and feel competent and confident to play.

But I haven't gone under, and I am grateful that I could leave them. I am on a lonely trip of self-discovery. I lived in six places last year. There were many times when I had nothing to give anyone.

How could I have done it? I ask myself as I sit alone in my cold, funky room. But I had to do what I did. I had to say yes to myself after so many of his no's, and my own too. Yes, there is a time when one must leave. For me it happened when a tiny whisper inside my chest became a shout I could no longer ignore. Yes, I left. But I sit here wondering, Are they wearing their gloves?

BARBARA N. BIDDLE is forty-two and was married for twenty-two years, during which time she mothered four children, served as Red Cross chairwoman, and was a columnist for a newspaper in New Hampshire.

Surviving, with a Little Help from My Daughters

LYNN GAIL

During July of 1975, I found myself facing life with my four-year-old daughter, Jennifer, my one-month-old infant, Joanna, and no husband. After eight years of marriage, my husband and I had decided to separate. For me, the separation initiated a period of intense pain and anger. My whole world — one that I had so carefully dreamed of and planned for, and that I had existed in during the marriage — fell apart, completely.

Because her father had moved across the country and had very little communication with his daughters, Jennifer was afraid that I too might leave her. I had to assure her continually that I would never leave her and that the divorce was not her fault. I explained to my daughter that her father and I could no longer live together as husband and wife in a good, healthy way, but that we would always be her mama and daddy.

Although a young child at that time, Jennifer knew me incredibly well. She had shared the rough periods during my married years and the pain of the actual break-up. She helped me to survive as a single mother just by caring for and loving me. She trusted me to keep the family together and to take good care of her and her sister. Jennifer and I became a team in a struggle for our lives. We kept our house a home. We served as supports, confidantes, and as outlets for our emotions — whether we were hugging, crying, or expressing anger. As mother and daughter, we were connected by feelings of loss, sadness, and anger. I needed her terribly.

Although my younger daughter was only a baby at the time of our separation, she also has been an important resource during the difficult five years of single motherhood. Her sweetness and tenderness have been a refreshing source of strength during these bittersweet years. Nursing and holding her, watching her grow and develop into herself, has been a wonderful experience. During tense times, the humorous and childlike interactions with Joanna helped Jennifer and me to laugh; we began to enjoy life as a family.

During the months immediately following the separation, I felt rage and chose to express it. I was furious with my ex-husband for deserting our family. I was also angry with myself for not creating a marriage that could "last forever," having believed that I could do so to such an extent that my whole world crumbled when the bubble burst.

Jennifer expressed her anger by refusing to really believe that our family of four — mother, father, big sister, and little sister — was gone and could never, ever be put back together. She continued to question me about whether or not I "hated" Daddy, or was still her friend, long after the divorce had been finalized. She was also hurt over her father's lack of communication with her.

We both released our anger physically by dancing, stretching, drawing, and punching pillows. We shared our expressions, thereby supporting each other's need to believe that it was all right to be sad and angry.

A nonverbal conversation and a closeness between mother and daughter, between friends, was developing. Later on, we were able to verbalize our feelings.

I felt terribly alone and frightened of facing my new singles world while taking care of my children. The evening hours at home were the most difficult for me. After the children were put to bed, too late for the phone to ring with a call from a friend, loneliness and sadness would haunt me. Tears would flow in rushes, finally expressing the fear and confusion of my life as a single mother, in financial debt, desperately trying to survive. When I became deeply depressed, and my frustration erupted into anger at my children, a pile of papers, a burned dinner, or anything, Jennifer would be there to support me. She would come over to me and stroke my hair slowly. She would hug and hold me, assuring me of her love. "Don't worry, Mama," she would say. "Everything will be all right. I'll help you."

Sometimes my life situation struck me as almost ludicrous: here I was feeling like a child and needing so much help, yet I was taking care of two children. Realistically, I had to be the strong, responsible adult. Fortunately, I could also be a child with Jennifer and Joanna.

I wanted to share the truth about my life with my children: I was a mother first, but also a friend to my daughters. Sometimes it became confusing as to where the boundaries lay, and I recognized a need for a balance. For example, I had to keep my disciplinary rules firm, but I also had to be open to the emotional needs of my children. Beds had to be straightened before breakfast, toys and clothes picked up, and no running or yelling was permitted in the house. There is security in knowing that things have to be done in certain ways. By structuring our lives with consistent limits, I was definitely the mother of the house. But the doorway for intimacy was also open, enabling us to be friends and our individual selves, as well as family members.

———————

One of the most difficult aspects of being a single parent was doing something for myself without feeling guilty that I was being selfish or a "bad" parent. I decided to attend graduate school in the expressive arts and then spent a great deal of time planning how my children would be taken care of while I was in school. I explained as honestly as possible my feelings that mothers have things they want and need to do. Because my daughters were already experiencing so many changes, I tried to be positive, sensitive, and strong when presenting any new developments in my life to them.

It was not easy to attend graduate school five days a week, drive close to an hour each way, be a mother to a five-year-old and a one-year-old, take care of the house, shop and cook, be a friend, and also be a single woman. Often I felt like a switchboard operator working with too many wires — plugging them in and out, hoping that all the connections would be made. Would Jennifer be left at kindergarten because my friend might forget to pick her up? Did I remember the car seat for the baby? Did I pay the baby sitter? Are all my notebooks for school in the orange bag? I needed to plan it out carefully so I could be comfortable each day and thus free enough to really get into the learning and processing at school.

———————

I had mixed feelings about motherhood after the divorce. I wanted to raise my children and have them live with me, but I also wanted to experience what other single women have the opportunity to live out. I discovered tremendous anger about not having that freedom. Legally I was a single woman; but I did not *feel* single. I always had my two children in my life. Then I would feel guilty. Was I a horrible mother to feel this way? Did any other single mothers have these thoughts? It was almost impossible to combine a single-type lifestyle with motherhood, and I needed to have both components in my life.

After my marriage broke up, I wondered if I could ever have a successful, long-lasting relationship with a man. I questioned whether I was attractive, sexual, sensual, or intelligent. I needed to find answers to these questions, so I began to establish a life outside my mother role. I had to become confident as a woman as well as a mother.

It felt strange to bring new men into the house. Jennifer would back off from them even in conversation. I projected her feelings and felt even more guilty that perhaps she resented me for replacing her father with new men.

Dating and time alone away from my children became expensive. I always had unpaid bills. As a single parent, I either had to take the children with me or pay for a sitter to watch them. Often I traded off with other single-parent friends, and this was wonderful.

Sometimes I hated my children for preventing me from leading a completely single life. I wished they would disappear. My dreams became nightmares of longing for freedom, yet wanting a deep, close relationship with my children as their mother. Sometimes I chose to be totally there for my children during the evening or on the weekends. Often I would go to bed at nine o'clock and wake up early on a weekend morning to have a long, relaxing breakfast with my daughters. Other times I would get a sitter and go out dancing with a friend, stay out until early morning, and sleep late the next day. I am still working out the balance between being a mother and a single woman.

I was not in any hurry to establish another relationship with a man. When I did have my space away from my children, I often chose to be by myself. Sometimes I wanted the company of my sister, a friend, or a small group of close friends. Having very confused feelings about myself with men, I felt more comfortable and relaxed with women. It has taken me five years to begin to establish a healthy relationship with a man.

Slowly my life is coming together. After being in financial debt for five years, I am finally stabilizing our finances so that we can live a simple but happy life.

Looking back, I am glad I shared all I did with my children. I did not create a Superwoman or Supermother role model for Jennifer and Joanna. They know me for who I am: a survivor.

LYNN GAIL is an expressive and movement therapist in the mental health and pediatric units of a hospital outside Boston. She also teaches at Tufts University and is writing a book.

14

*Becoming
a Stepmother*

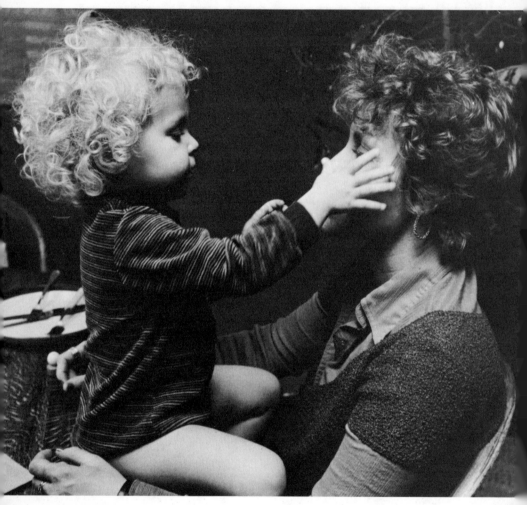

Gail LeBoff

Front-Seat Politics

LEE F. GRUZEN

One June afternoon, seven years ago, I met Alex — a compact, blond eleven-year-old — fast asleep in the front seat of his father's car. My romance with his father, Jordan, was only a month old, but already charmed. I had primed myself for a momentous meeting with my stepson-to-be.

Never having been a parent, I didn't know what to expect. But I thought, somehow, that there would be a magical moment when Alex and I would feel related and loving, as if by instinct. After all, chances were good that the word *mother* would be part of my new title, along with *wife*.

But my feelings weren't tender, and the meeting wasn't dramatic. I sized him up: cute, but too big to be adorable, straightforward, easy to talk with, gentle, and mature. In fact, he seemed too mature, too self-assured; he struck me as a personality to be reckoned with. Instantly I claimed *my* front seat and moved him to the back where children belong.

We did find our special shared moment later, when it was time to decide where to eat a late lunch. Alex and I happened to nominate the same favorite Chinese restaurant, a place unknown to Jordan. That simple coincidence, the day's only magic, delighted both Alex and me, and throughout the afternoon we chatted easily about life in the sixth grade, the dangers of monosodium glutamate, and our excellent taste in food. I even started imagining our annual Chinatown reunion.

Since then, the same disparate emotions of that first encounter have been repeated again and again. My rivalry and irritation with Alex surface regularly. The preordained, automatic, unquestioning love between a mother and son simply is not there. What we do have has been slowly created by connections as small, human, and unexpected as the choice of the same Szechuan restaurant.

Jordan and I were together for three years before we were married, and Alex spent most every weekend and vacation with us, except for six weeks when he left for summer camp. Otherwise he lived with his mother and his future stepfather.

I complained endlessly to Jordan about our lack of free time alone together, especially on Friday nights and the dreadful first days of vacation trips when I was always tired, anxious, and desperate to find peace of mind. With Alex around there would be intermittent squabbling, usually provoked by my compulsive need to criticize and put him in his place whenever possible. Never noticing our quick and subtle skirmishes, Jordan thought our time together was always calm and enjoyable, with or without Alex. But I knew the difference. Alone with Jordan I had harmony, romance, and the reassurance of his single-minded attention; and after all, it was with Jordan, not Alex, that I had chosen to spend my time.

Nevertheless, Jordan and Alex were accustomed to their seven-year routine, dating back to Jordan's divorce, and the patterns were too fixed and cherished to be changed. I resented the history they had shared without me and felt imposed upon; but it was impossible not to respect Jordan for his steady caring for his son. I carped, and he ignored me.

On a typically bad Friday night, the three of us would head for Long Island to visit Jordan's parents, who would dote on Alex, promising him a horse when he turned thirteen and praising him for his cooking (when I had been the one to shop, chop, and clean up for his messy extravaganzas). They would laugh off his nonstop noisy television watching, even though it drove the rest of us from the tiny house, and they would listen adoringly to his precocious analysis of mathematical formulas and submarine designs. I knew, of course, that Alex was getting only what he deserved from an appreciative family that encouraged his talents, but the fact that my resentments were unjust only made matters worse.

My ego was extremely fragile at that time. When I first met Jordan I was finishing up a two-year stretch as a cable television producer with a nonprofit company. I was ready for "big-time" network television, but the transition took well over a year, with at least fifty interviews and two periods of unemployment. I was also straining to adjust to Jordan's style of living. He was thirty-nine and a well-known New York architect, with older friends, sophisticated tastes, and a calendar filled with social events. Jobless and twenty-seven, I was insecure about clothes, savoir faire, you name it. No wonder Alex's power bothered me. At thirteen he was the confident kid in control of his universe, the big cheese, the star. He was everything that I wanted to be.

When one hundred people celebrated his bar mitzvah and his "manhood," I became miserably jealous. I still didn't think of myself as a full-fledged woman. How dare he consider himself anything but a boy?

Yet Alex and I did get along well much of the time, particularly when the two of us shared something which Jordan wasn't part of, like singing Judy Collins's version of "Amazing Grace," rating Barry Manilow's new records, or mugging for the camera on top of a Cape Cod sand dune.

There were sixteen years between the two of us, but when we talked about music we seemed close in age, ganging up on Jordan to switch the radio from the classical to the rock stations. When I went to work for NBC shows that he liked to watch, Alex cheered and boasted about my job to his friends.

Alex also flattered me in odd, improbable ways. He brought his mother to meet me two weeks after our Chinese lunch. Year after year he wore the "Today Show" T-shirt I'd scrounged up for him. He thought the first spaghetti I cooked for him, a single glutinous wad, was the funniest thing he'd ever seen. While skiing he patiently waited for me at numerous chilly stops along the mountain. He even willingly packed my books the day I moved in with his father. On our first boat trip together, he awakened me for help after throwing up — one of the few times I've truly felt like his mother.

After Jordan and I married, Alex transferred to a high school in our neighborhood and began spending more time with us. Cold war broke out over the issue of territory: our bedroom. Alex had his own room and black-and-white television. But I had the color set *and* the cable hook-up with the movie channel *and* the upstairs phone. Alex had been camping out there for years before me, and he felt justified in stretching out on my bed or popping in and out to answer calls from his teenage friends. In a new marriage, a strange

235

apartment, and a hectic job, I felt desperate for a "room of my own" in which to calm down and relax. The bedroom symbolized the only place where I might find peace. My desk, books, and special objects were there, and although I shared it with Jordan, the bedroom was intended to be my safe, nourishing space.

On Friday nights, Alex would come home, exuberantly chatting about his week. For me he was an occupier, an intruder, an uncontrolled enemy, and I would greet him icily. We regularly discussed my feelings and just as regularly he would then humbly ask to come in. This only made matters more frustrating, because I could never say no to him when he presented a logical argument, which was always. His occupation of our room to watch a ninety-minute replay of *Yellow Submarine* in color seemed more valuable than my locking myself in the same room to read a book that I could read elsewhere. But for months at a time I was too angry to look him fully in the face.

It actually took years to resolve the conflict. Bribing Alex with a color television set on his sixteenth birthday helped. Support from my friends about the validity of my need for a personal space was crucial. Most important, Alex gradually became more active socially on weekends and didn't want to hang around with us as much. Life improved.

Alex's mother's frankness and feedback were invaluable. She told me that she too had kicked him out of her room, that many times when he returned home she also resented his intrusion; most important, she said that Alex liked me and was not suffering from my stormy attacks. Tactfully she reminded me that Alex had two accessible parents whom he adored, grandparents nearby, and reasonable stepparents with whom he got along well. His psyche and sense of himself were strong and resilient and not about to be tumbled by me. According to her, my effect on him was positive. In other words, she gave me permission to tell him off when I needed to and not to feel like a rat for doing so.

If, in fact, she were less of a presence in her son's life, I might feel more like his mother, with a starring role and clear, satisfying responsibilities. Instead I'm a member of Alex's supporting cast, and I think that she, also a stepmother, knows that the second-fiddle part takes getting used to.

───────────

When my daughter Rachel was born, our household changed dramatically. Alex became the big brother, taking care of the baby, showing her off, and delighting in her first word, "Ali." He cross-country skiied through Central Park with Rachel in his backpack, to introduce her to his buddies, and brought her replicas of his own old favorite toys.

He announced regularly that he, like Rachel, had been a chubby, blond baby. But because of his fifteen-year advantage, his overall maturity, and Jordan's style of fathering, Alex's jealousy of Rachel seemed nonexistent. For his senior class yearbook he chose a jubilant photograph of Rachel and him, side by side, on their first day of school.

Rachel also afforded a showcase for Alex's developing personality. His patience, levelheadedness, physical strength, warmth, and steadiness became valuable to Rachel and me, and we needed him. He kept her company when Jordan and I traveled. When last spring's family outing on steep mountains became treacherous, he carried her to safety. He even protected us during the summers, when I'd be nervous about staying without Jordan in the country. I grew to respect him in a new way.

My relationship with Alex has also improved because I've become far more comfortable in my roles as wife, mother, working woman, and stepmother. Less touchy, insecure, and muddled about my life, I no longer resent Alex's success or worry about controlling him. I'm finally able to communicate grievances directly rather than sideways by innuendo. He and I have also resolved a few old issues. He stays clear of my bedroom, keeps silent about his mother's great food, eats snacks willingly to keep alive until our late dinners, and doesn't ask to tag along on spring vacations. He also leaves the front seat to me, unless he's driving. And then I'm thrilled that he takes the wheel so I can snooze and daydream.

In exchange, I cook his favorite foods, remember the sour cream for his baked potatoes, offer advice on his clothes only when asked, share the cable television occasionally, and welcome him warmly on Christmas and summer vacations. We accept and enjoy our own spheres of influence.

Of course our genuinely friendly accommodation does not mean that I won't rage at him over other violations: beating his father at sports; lecturing me on my lifestyle; leaving dirty dishes in the sink; and assuming that he should be free to read the morning paper while I cook his eggs.

I am certain that my deep-seated and poorly understood rivalries with my younger brother affect my relationship with Alex, making me more prone to compete with him for attention and also arousing in me an old, familiar guilt. Fortunately, Alex also benefits from the love I have for my brother, and I often use their names interchangeably.

Alex is now getting ready for a summer hosteling trip abroad, to be followed by college. To my surprise, I regret his leaving. Not that I'll miss playing stepmother — that role never felt authentic. I'm still too young, and he'll always be too old for that. But I enjoy being Alex's older stepsister, and I'd even consider surrendering my front seat if he would stay on.

LEE F. GRUZEN was a production associate, researcher, and producer with documentary film and television companies for ten years before she became a mother at thirty-two. She is currently living in Manhattan and writing a monthly movie review for a small New York City magazine.

No Difference in Degree

ANNE T. JACKSON

I took the steps two at a time. I knew when I got to the fourth floor, I'd be breathless and therefore speechless. I must have wanted to arrive that way. Physically and figuratively, I was rushing up toward my unknown future. I was frightened — about to meet Victoria, aged sixteen, who was soon to become my stepdaughter.

As I burst through the door, I saw her at once, sitting absolutely still, facing me. We looked directly at each other. Her whole body gave a kind of quick start; she said nothing.

What I saw was a beautiful young woman. What I sensed was an intelligent, sensitive, angry, lonely girl who adored her handsome, dynamic father so much that she had found enough courage to meet me in a civilized, polite manner. And she was, I sensed, more frightened than I.

I wanted to tell her I was not her enemy, nor was I her rival coming to take away her father's love. I wanted to tell her all the things I sensed about her, and that if we could find the ways to help one another, things would get better, not worse. But I said none of those things because I knew that from her view of life, I was her enemy. I knew too that only time could help us. It did.

All those momentary, fleeting realizations overwhelmed me, but they also changed something: I ceased to fear my future role as stepmother. I had a clear prescience that I would never be expected to be, in the traditional sense, a mother. That realization was to be a key to our future relations and was for me a great relief.

I genuinely like children and always have. But even with my own, whom I love more deeply than anything on earth, I never have been the stereotypical "motherly-mother." I have worked, almost continuously, since I was sixteen. I've always believed in what we now call "children's rights." I see no reason why *my* children should naturally like what I like, think the way I do, have the same talents, fears, or habits. If they do, fine. If they don't, then it makes our interactions that much more diverse and interesting.

At some level I wish to extend my sense of independence to others, because I believe no one owns another. We are all alone. If, as Shakespeare wrote, "The truth [I] speak doth lacke some gentleness," I respond that within our abilities we can only try to help one another. Sometimes we succeed; sometimes we agonize over failure; the failures make us feel guilty.

I was thirty-eight when I became stepmother to Ron's three children: Victoria, then sixteen; David, fourteen; and Peter, five. I had been separated and divorced for two years, and my sons — Jack, sixteen; Michael, fourteen; and Simon, nine — had been living with me and visiting their father whenever they or he wished. At the time I had an intellectually stimulating job which I enjoyed greatly, and I intended to continue working.

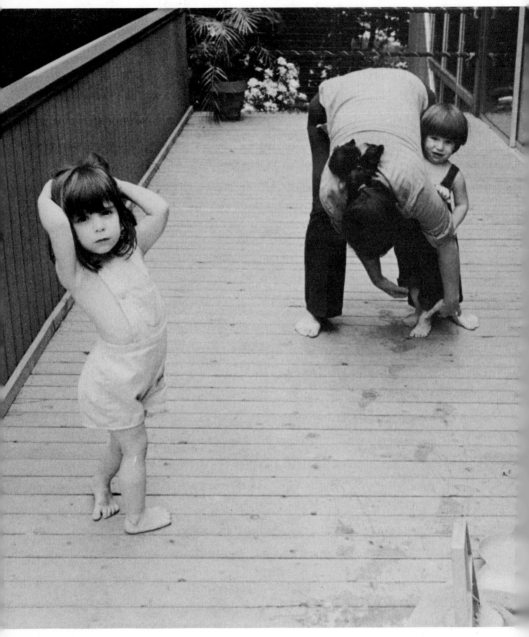

Gail LeBoff

Like every divorced parent, I felt guilty over the failure of my first marriage, most especially as it affected my children. But they were healthy and normally bright; they were loved and loving, and the energy that bounced back and forth between us bred only optimism.

How did I feel about being a stepmother?

After that first encounter with Victoria, I felt hopeful, and after meeting charming, happy-go-lucky David, I felt very good. My feelings about Peter, the baby of the family, were another matter. He was a shrill, nervous, bright child, who for years behaved like the spoiled brat he was. It took us years to become friends. But I was so happy to be marrying Ron, whom I passionately loved, that I did not feel dreary about the future as a stepmother.

Ron's children had been living far away with their mother for about three years. He either visited them every few weeks, or they came to stay with him. But he missed them terribly, and on top of that he felt guilty over not being a full-time father. We hoped that Ron's two oldest children would come to live with us, and within a year this came about.

From the beginning of our marriage, Ron was wonderful with my sons. He did all he could to make them feel secure and loved. He was their friend, and in time they came to know it. But initially my two oldest sons regarded him as their enemy. The anger they felt toward me and the new man in my life showed itself in the usual adolescent behavior, but all our emotional reactions were unusually intense.

Some of the displays were amusing. I remember one evening, while I was preparing dinner, I heard Ron ask sixteen-year-old Jack to set the table, something I often asked of him and which he would do without any fuss. Jack said, "O.K.," but did nothing. After a few minutes, I quietly asked him again. Nothing. Just as the meal was ready to be served, Jack proceeded, at top speed, to get out the "best" dishes, glassware, and cutlery. This was not easy to do and was hair-raising to watch because I kept all my precious "best" on the highest, most child-proof closet shelves, and I did *not* use them for everyday family eating. Naturally, I yelled. Jack argued. Ron and the others joined the scene — expecting to eat. They found me furious, a partylike table half-laid, and Jack, smug as a cat, calmly pretending innocence, obedience, and accomplishment.

The problem was that when my children upset me, Ron became upset with them, which in turn caused me to be upset for both Ron and the children. I knew Jack knew this; he had baited the hook, and I had swallowed it. It was Ron's sense of humor that broke the tension. He said it was time we ate from decent dishes; who was I saving them for? He then told several jokes about people doing clumsy things. It was hard not to laugh, so we did. In those early days, it was often Ron's wittiness that diffused the anger, and in time I learned not to bite at the bait so quickly.

————————

The turning point at which we all began to interact like a real family came months later, during our first summer vacation. We rented a large lakeside house and had all six of our children together for a month, for the first time.

It was an extraordinary experience. It was hellish and it was heavenly. It was the best and worst of times, and for me it was certainly no vacation.

What we did and said and how we interacted as a family somehow unlocked our emotions, both happy and unhappy ones, and we began to get a good and realistic look at one another.

There were quarrels among the children, scenes between Ron and me, minor accidents, fraternal friendships begun, and many triumphs: Peter learned to swim; Simon learned to water-ski the first time he tried; Victoria fell in love (it was then that she and I began to trust and love one another); Jack wrote a play and gave every child for miles around a part in it; Michael, to his surprise, became a star pitcher and idol of the baseball set; and David developed a psychic knack for finding, and bringing home, huge fish which no one wanted to scale, let alone clean or eat. There were boat rides, picnics, moonlight swimming parties, card games, and mountains of food.

I remember thinking about my own mother. How would she have coped with this gang? When I was little, she told me how she had always dreamed of having four sons and two daughters, whereas she had only my brother and me. Although we always had a tribe of friends at our house, it hardly prepared me for my current role. For one thing, unlike my mother, I had never been particularly interested in cooking, nor was I fussy about food. My children were used to this, and they would either eat what I gave them or get themselves something else. Not so my stepchildren. To them food was a thrill. They had passionate likes and dislikes, not necessarily the same from day to day. But when one liked something, he or she plowed in, and the rest of us had to be very deft, or vociferous, or go hungry.

During that vacation I began to realize, for the first time in my life, that my indifferent cooking efforts were not necessarily acceptable. Because I had the time, I tried a little harder. No one noticed or appreciated it any better; I began to resent the time I spent; I openly resented and responded to further criticism, and then, when my own kids, in a rush of general agreement, told me what a lousy cook I was, I wept outwardly and raged inwardly. Ron, bless him, defended my culinary skills and announced that he would not tolerate any more nonsense. After that, everyone made tentative and then fiercely snide jokes about my efforts, but they ate the food and stopped complaining about it.

Yes, in those early days I often felt harassed, overworked, misunderstood, angry with myself and others, and I worried about events over which I had no control. With all that, though, slowly, slowly, I came to know my stepchildren. We carefully tested one another, we respected one another, we learned to trust one another, and our liking slowly turned to love. It did not happen all at once or quickly. What did happen almost instantly, and in a way it was both remarkable and probably responsible for the closeness we all have today, was that my children and stepchildren became closest friends — brothers-to-brothers, sister-to-brothers. There is little doubt that they helped one another get over the problems of divorce. To this day, with most of them married and some with children of their own, all far away and busy with their lives, they still care deeply for one another.

Accepting the fact that I was a "lousy" cook was just one lesson I learned. In a small way, it illustrates the core of the problem of stepfamilies: getting to know all those peculiar, little things about one another and then accepting or rejecting the knowledge; getting to know oneself through another's eyes and, equally important, either accepting or rejecting that knowledge.

There are two things that every member of our combined family has helped me to learn. First, that truth is an abstraction which has many facets; and second, that the emotion we call love has more facets than a million jewels.

These are the greatest gifts I have ever received. They have enabled me to feel and to say that the kind of love I have for *my* stepchildren is no different in degree from the kind of love I feel for my *husband's* stepchildren. This did not come easily or quickly. I experienced harrowing times — one son in jail for drug abuse; a stepson who dropped out; and a resurrection by sons and stepsons. But we never divided ourselves as children versus stepchildren, or as parent versus stepparent. We worked out our problems as a family. I never attempted to be a mother to my stepchildren. But I did work at creating a cohesive family, one whose members understand and accept one another.

Once upon a time I was introduced in this way: ". . . and, er, this is my father's wife." And once upon a better time I was introduced in this way: "This is my stepmother." And that *is* a difference in degree.

ANNE T. JACKSON is a nom de plume. The author was born in the United Kingdom. She has worked as a dancer, journalist, editor, and director of publications in law, education, medicine, and computer science.

15

*Foster, Adoptive,
and Natural Mothers*

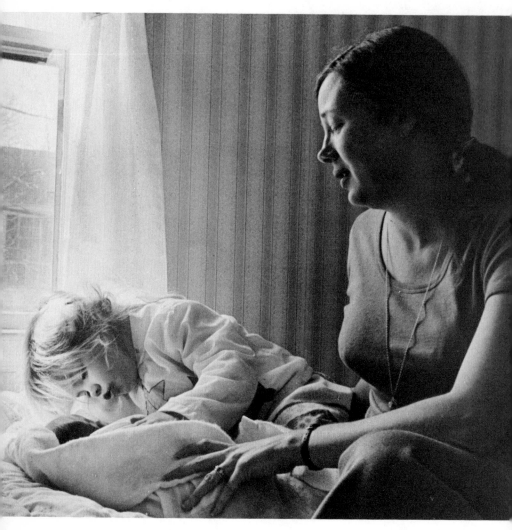

Alice Moulton

Not flesh of my flesh
Nor bone of my bone
But, yet, miraculously,
My own.

Don't forget
Not for a minute
You weren't born under my heart
But in it.

— Anonymous

The Fostering of Tammy and Danielle

M. R. LAMB

September 1977, *High Noon.* I am nervously pacing about the living room. I pass by the mirror and look at myself: thirty-nine years old, shortly to turn forty, still small and trim, with red hair that is always a bit too fluffy. Small lines are starting to wind their way around my eyes. There is still a hint of youth, but there is also a mature serenity about my expression. My fears of post-hysterectomy atrophy have been totally dispelled by what I see in my reflection. Suddenly my thoughts are interrupted by the clamor at the front door. When I open it, I will become a new mother once again — the foster mother of two infant daughters.

I yank open the heavy old door to admit the two social workers, each clutching a thin, shabbily dressed infant in one arm and a shopping bag in the other. My heart swells and tears fill my eyes from the pitiful sight before me. I shut the door, leading social workers with babies and shopping bags to the sofa. I press myself into its comfortable fold, trying to absorb as much data as I can on the backgrounds of these children, "my" foster children.

They have arrived from the hospital after extensive treatment for severe malnutrition and failure to thrive. I cannot imagine that what I am seeing is real. These babies sit before me frail and vulnerable, perhaps even brain damaged. All my fears and doubts about fostering a child vanish and are replaced by love and determination. My heart says, Now you are mine, although perhaps not forever. For the time that we do have together, we will love, we will laugh, we will cry, and we will grow as a family.

I take a child into each arm, and kiss them. They respond to me, each cuddling against my breast. I feel exactly as I did each time I had delivered and my newborn lay quietly against me, a beautiful and cherished moment. I had never dreamed that I would again experience that moment, and yet I feel it now. I enjoy my inner bliss but also attempt to listen to the information coming from the social workers.

Tammy is twenty months old and does not crawl, stand, talk, or laugh. She rarely cries and has seldom been out of her crib.

Danielle is six months old and cannot roll over or sit up. From constantly lying in one position in her crib, she is totally bald on the back of her head. She is thought to be retarded due to prolonged malnutrition.

I should feel hopeless and depressed, given how grim it all sounds. I can already hear the negative comments from my family and friends: "Don't you think that you're taking on too much? How can you hope to accomplish very much with these children? Your own children will be jealous of the extra attention Tammy and Danielle will require."

Well, I'll simply have to ignore everyone and their opinions if I'm going to make this work, and work it must to ensure that these babies have a happy, healthy, loving childhood. I'm determined and I know that somehow I can do it.

Christmas Morning, 1977. My five older children, ranging from thirteen to nineteen, are all fast asleep. I'm so pleased with their love and understanding for Tammy and Danielle. They are constantly attentive to the little ones' wants and needs. I have their unanimous approval and support, and the progress being made is now a team effort. I listen at the stairway and I can hear Tammy calling out, "Momma." Yes, she now has a two-word vocabulary, consisting of *momma* and *baby*. She also walks and laughs. I am terribly proud of each of her accomplishments, however small some might seem.

My husband, Leonard, is helping me bathe the babies this morning so that we can get dinner organized. It's so much fun for us to be back to the baby-bathing routine after such a long hiatus. I look at him from the side and notice his double chin, matched by his rounded belly. His temples are graying, and he, too has those little lines around his deep-set brown eyes. I love him even more today than I did twenty years ago. He praises me for the amazing progress that Tammy and Danielle have made. I glow, and when I glance into the mirror of late, I see a more youthful reflection.

Danielle, who can now sit up regally, splashes at the bath with great gusto, soaking everything within a five-foot radius. (It's a great way to keep the dust down.) I look at their once emaciated bodies and smile at the sight of their now chubby faces and bottoms, with fingers and toes like tight sausages extending from rounded arms and legs. I'm protective and possessive. I suddenly am reminded of the reality that they are not my own. One day I will have to give them up. I push that idea aside, as I cannot stand to think of it. This is one problem no one can help me with. I should deal with it realistically and face the inevitable future, yet I dismiss it totally from my mind. How will I handle something I cannot even bear to think about? Perhaps that day of parting will never come to be.

Thanksgiving Day, 1978. I have been a mother for twenty years now. It is beautiful to see so many young people seated around the dining room table. It's been a wonderful year of growth and development for Tammy and Danielle. Tammy is a bright, energetic toddler. She is verbally slow, but we are working with her and

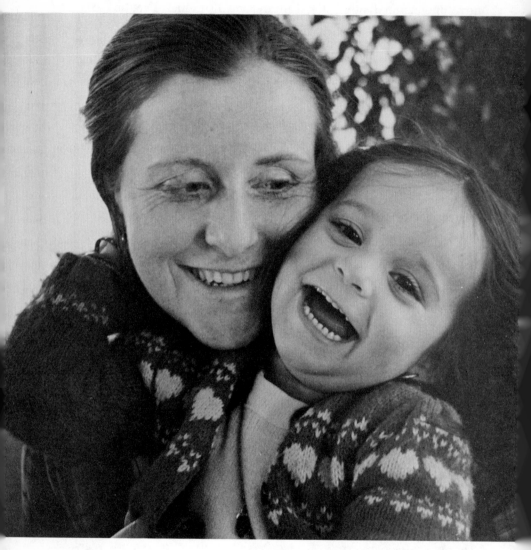

Margaret Thompson

believe that she soon will be speaking more fluently. Danielle is marvelous and ahead of herself in all aspects of development. I did it. No, *we* did it, with patience and trusting love. I feel so good about myself. I was able to give, share, and love so deeply that all the obstacles in my way disappeared one by one. I still have a great fear of the inevitable separation, yet I am unable to consider it as a reality. I should, I must, I will — perhaps tomorrow. Today is just too wonderful.

March 1979. My world is shattering. Leonard is in the cardiac intensive unit. I left the babies in the charge of the older children and begin the ordeal of waiting. I've spent so many days of my life waiting in hospitals for "the news," sometimes good and other times bad. Because of my medical professional background it should be easier for me. Yet the tension of the unknown is unbearable. Leonard and I have always waited together. Now I must wait alone, cry alone, think alone.

Leonard has not felt well for some time. The years of commuting to work each day, the business trips and flight connections, the never-ending house repairs, and the emotional and financial responsibilities of a large and growing family have taken their toll. He deserves much more time. We all need and love him so dearly. We'll reorganize our lives and make all the necessary adjustments, if he'll just get well.

Summer 1979. Our lives are changing to a slower, more relaxed pace. While some changes come with ease, others are terribly painful and difficult: Tammy and Danielle are going through an adoptive process. Because of our age and Leonard's heart condition, we are not adoptive candidates.

Finally comes the inevitable parting that I have avoided for two years. I cannot imagine life without my Tammy and Danielle. I wonder if they can imagine life without me. We are mutually in love, we three, and I cry myself to sleep at night. I know that they will go to a fine couple who will want and love them as much as we have. But will they feel so rejected that they suffer psychologically? Will they grow up hating the mother who gave them away?

The social worker has given me a tentative departure date. I cherish every moment of every day that we have left together.

Summer drifts lazily into a crisp fall season. Halloween is peeking around the corner again, and this year Tammy and Danielle will don the traditional spook paraphernalia, thus commencing the ritual "trick or treat." The state, with its never-ending red tape and delays, has given us more time to be together. I'm selfishly pleased, although the delays are not beneficial for the children. The older they get, the more difficult it will be for them to leave us. They are so delighted by piles of leaves, busy chattering squirrels, and smiling pumpkins. They renew for me wonderful, faraway memories.

———————

Christmas Eve, 1979. This will be our third and final Christmas together in the big old house. Tammy and Danielle have napped this afternoon, because Santa is coming to see them this evening. Leonard is poised with the camera, and everyone is alert with anticipation.

The sliding door opens and in he comes. In all my life, I will never forget their blue eyes and baby smiles of sheer delight at the vision of Santa. He is complete with a small sack of toys and two large rocking horses. The room is tumultuous. The flashes are popping, and the evening proceeds as I drift away nostalgically through all the past Christmases. This is truly the best, but I feel an overwhelming sadness at the finality of it. What will it be like next Christmas? Quiet and lonely.

———————

January 1980, *High Noon*. I close the heavy living room door. I watch, through tear-filled eyes, as Tammy and Danielle and part of me leave forever. It is noon once again, and as I pass the old mirror, I hesitate. Look at yourself. Look at the past two-and-a-half years beaming at you. Dry your eyes. Don't be sad. So much of life is a brief encounter. You of all people should understand: you will cry; you will laugh; you will be lonely; and you will be fulfilled. Most of all, you will remember, and you will never be forgotten!

———————

To My Beloved Foster Daughters

You're leaving soon
I have such emotion
Dealing with this.

You're leaving soon
No longer will I hear
Your footsteps each morn
Clambering down the hallway.
You're leaving soon
No longer will I hear
Your ever-changing voices
Calling out, "Hi Mom."
You're leaving soon
No longer will I see
Your bright, happy faces
Coming round the corner stair.

You're leaving soon
And I shall stare
At empty hall and wall and stair
And I will care
And for all eternity, each time
I round the corner stair —
I shall see you both,

      Smiling there.

M. R. LAMB is a pen name the author uses in memory of her second son, who died at the age of three of congenital birth defects. She lives in Boston.

Not Flesh of My Flesh

CAROLYN JACOBS

I am an infertile mother. I have experienced the ultimate in depression during long years of doctors' visits and infertility testing, and I have experienced the ultimate in joy when we were able to adopt two healthy infants. As I sit here trying to write during the brief snatches of time when my children are sleeping and there are no pressing emergencies, I know full well how blessed I am. My life for the past few years has been an emotional roller coaster, going from frustration to fulfillment, from despondency to delight, from pessimism to optimism. My house has gone from neat and serene to a place cluttered with toys and filled with the excited squeals of young children. I'm half as organized, but twice as happy.

When we decided we were ready to have children, Eric and I had been married for five years, with good, secure jobs, a new four-bedroom house, and no inkling in the world that filling up the spare bedrooms would be the most trying, difficult, and divisive time of our married life.

Eight months after I'd stopped taking birth-control pills I first spoke to my gynecologist about the possibility of infertility, and six months later I was under the care of one of the best-known endocrinologists and infertility specialists in Philadelphia.

The initial infertility testing was, at least, bearable, since there was a need to diagnose what was keeping me from conceiving. Each test brought to light some problem which, if taken by itself, could easily be overcome, but when combined with many others, seemed to be insurmountable. There was never a conclusive diagnosis of infertility in our case, and for years we held out hope that some combination of drugs or treatments just might do the trick. I would sit and listen disconsolately as my doctor explained how little was really known about infertility, and how endocrinology was like a jigsaw puzzle — you had to keep trying things to see if all the pieces might fit together. As the years passed, so did my optimism.

The testing turned out to be disastrous to our sex life. We almost always had "sex on schedule," because the temperature chart or the doctor's office demanded it, and we almost never had intercourse for the fun or mutual satisfaction of it. Even now, more than two years after we stopped treatments, we haven't regained the spontaneity and enthusiasm we had before sex became a necessary chore.

To explain my frequent absences from work, occasioned by the testing and treatments, I suddenly developed (as far as my boss and colleagues were concerned) a chronically sore back, terrible teeth and gum problems, a car that gave me nothing but trouble, and numerous viral infections. I hated myself for being devious, yet I couldn't admit to anyone in my office that I was undergoing infertility testing.

I was working as a senior-level computer system designer at the time, and was a prime candidate for advancement into a managerial position. Instead of aggressively seeking such a position (which would normally have been in my nature to do), I shrank from the responsibility and began undermining my own career with a series of poor job decisions. I avoided long-range commitments and languished in one dead-end assignment after another. My job, which should have been an outlet for me, became instead a dreaded chore. I would daydream endlessly at work about what my new life would be like after I had a baby. I imagined people's reactions to the announcement that I'd be leaving, tried to figure out who would be planning my baby shower, and wrote lists of baby names instead of computer design documentation.

Each month would bring the fervent hope that the current treatment would be effective, and then the onset of my period would bring a crushing letdown. I would cry for hours — sometimes alone, sometimes with Eric — but always as though my problem were the worst in the world. I think now that I was actually in a prolonged state of mourning, grieving for the child I would never have. I felt morose most of the time, bored with everything, and restless to resolve my fate or have it resolved for me. I knew I needed some help to get me over my inertia and force me to plan positively for a possibly childless future, but I found no one to whom I could turn. My endocrinologist was totally unprepared and unwilling to deal with the emotional aspects of infertility and seemed completely insensitive as I sat sobbing before him. He suggested private counseling, but it was hard enough to deal with the high cost of our treatments, let alone afford any additional expenses. I felt totally alone.

Whenever I heard that a friend or acquaintance was pregnant I would explode in anger, not because I didn't want happiness for her, but because I was irrationally and insanely jealous. I began avoiding pregnant women because I didn't want to hear how they felt. It seemed, in my state of mind, that pregnancy was the only thing that pregnant women could talk about.

Next I began avoiding people with small children because the last thing I wanted was to be reminded of what I was missing. I even began ignoring the birth announcements that came in the mail because shopping for baby presents was too painful. More than once I found myself retreating into the ladies' room at work to cry because a conversation about pregnancy, delivery, or babies was more than I could bear.

I did share my feelings and experiences with a few of my very closest friends because I desperately needed confidantes. But as they conceived children and went to extremes to avoid telling me their news, I finally began to realize how difficult I was making it for my friends to deal with me. I didn't really like unburdening myself to others, and I was torn between wanting my friends to understand me yet wanting them not to pity me.

I look back on that period of my life with some feelings of shame. I was never able to come to grips successfully with the reality of my inability to bear children. I let my frustration affect almost every aspect of my life, from my job to my relationships with friends. Even now I find it difficult to face some of the people I once snubbed when I couldn't deal with their childbearing. And I've never been able to apologize, because I don't like to admit my shame and I'm afraid that others just won't understand the turmoil I was going through at the time.

———

Eric, my rock and my strong shoulder on which to cry, became an even greater source of frustration for me as time wore on. I wanted to adopt a baby, and he did not. I couldn't contemplate childlessness, and he could. He had serious doubts about his ability to love an adopted child and cherished fantasies about the high expectations he would have had for our natural-born child. He understood, appreciated, and sympathized with my desperate need, but it took months of soul-searching, crying together, and finally counseling to get him to agree to begin the process of finding a baby to adopt. He finally came to understand that we could have no guarantees of the beauty or intelligence of our own children, and that it was perfectly acceptable for him to agree to adopt while still maintaining his reservations and skepticism. It did not help my frustration level at all when each of the many sources we contacted was pessimistic about our chances of finding an available baby.

In the end, we were much luckier than most couples who adopt. We had (coincidentally) only nine months to wait until we got the phone call that said a newborn girl could be ours.

We celebrated the fulfillment of our dream with giddy laughter, excited whooping, and mild panic over how to prepare for her arrival. By now, Eric was as thrilled as I was. I could never adequately describe what we felt the day the baby arrived. The cliché, "the longest day of our lives," hardly comes close to depicting what our wait was like. Our baby was being brought to us from another state, and there were constant gnawing worries about whether the birth mother's resolve to carry through with the adoption had changed; whether the hospital release had gone smoothly; whether plane connections had been made; and, finally, what could possibly be taking so long. We sat for hours in our lawyer's house trying to find distractions from our fear and anticipation. I thought that the sound of the car doors slamming would scarcely be heard above the sound of my pounding heart.

The nurse who supervised the transfer handed the baby to us and had the good sense to leave us alone literally to cry our eyes out together. The three of us wailed, Eric and I from relief and elation, Lisa from hunger and fatigue. We drove home shakily with our most precious cargo, tenderly placed her in her crib, and stared in wonder. I remember a night filled with tears of gratitude, little sleep, and countless trips into her room just to be sure that she was still there.

A close friend called a few days later and asked, "Do you love her yet?" After some time, I answered, "No, I don't think I feel any special attachment to her yet." I agonized over that answer, worrying about what might be wrong with me after all the years of wanting so badly to have a child to love. I cannot tell you exactly when I truly felt love for her. I suspect it developed slowly over the first few weeks. I know that by the time she started smiling at me I felt not only love, but adulation.

When the exhilaration of the first few days wore off and I had some time to consider what had happened to me, I began to worry about the fact that someone else had a legal claim on Lisa. I would be awakened by nightmares about the knock on the door that meant she could be taken away from us. I tried very hard to imagine what it must have been like for the young girl who had given birth to her and then gave her away. I began to feel very grateful that in an age where the options of birth control and abortion both exist, she had chosen neither.

My early worries over losing Lisa were gradually replaced by new ones. I was frightened that the state agency which supervised our adoption would find something wrong with our home environment and recommend that the baby be placed elsewhere. I had heard horror stories that some illegalities in the transfer process had caused the courts to take a baby away from its adoptive parents. Once we'd passed the legal hurdles, undergone two court hearings, and had before us a birth certificate with Lisa's new name on it, a great burden of doubt and uncertainty was lifted.

As Lisa grows, talks, and understands more, I'm beginning to worry about the time she will realize what the word *adoption* means. The question, "Why did you adopt me?" has direct, easy answers; but I don't know how I'll be able to deal with, "Why didn't my birth mother want me?" I hope that Eric and I can make her understand that the environment that is now shaping her personality is vastly more important than the one that first shaped her body. I hope too that we can provide her with a secure-enough upbringing so that she will never feel the need to search for her birth parents, so that she can accept our roots as her very own. I want to be totally honest with her about the circumstances of her birth and adoption.

———————

I don't think Lisa is treated any differently from other children because she is adopted. I know that she is never taken for granted. Even when she is being obstreperous, cantankerous, recalcitrant, and typically two-year-old, she is deeply loved. Months and months go by sometimes when the events and feelings associated with her adoption never cross my mind. They don't seem particularly relevant to our relationship right now. I have learned to accept it as absolutely normal and perfectly natural when strangers tell me how much she resembles me. After all, Lisa is *our* daughter. There will never be any question about that in our minds and, I hope, not in hers either.

For a very short while after Lisa's arrival, I felt a bit sorry for myself because I would never experience a pregnancy — never feel the changes in my body, never feel a fetus kicking inside me, never feel and see my baby being born, and never nurse. I know, however, that as wonderful, awesome, and exhilarating as pregnancy may be, it is still only a means of attaining the ultimate objective of having a child to love, to raise, and with whom to share a life.

This past summer, two-and-a-half years after the miracle of Lisa, we were given the chance to adopt another baby girl. Although Deborah's arrival wasn't fraught with the same anxieties and excitement as Lisa's, she is just as wondrous and precious — a little icing on our beautiful family cake.

CAROLYN JACOBS worked for eleven years as a programmer, systems analyst, and systems designer before adopting her first daughter. She is from Cherry Hill, New Jersey.

Nursing an Adopted Child

GLORIA BENNETT

While I was growing up, I never gave much thought to the mechanics of having and caring for my future children. Because my mother had a child when I was eleven years old, I had plenty of experience with an infant. My baby brother and the young cousins born at this time in my life were all bottle-fed, and I never considered any other method of feeding. I can vividly remember during my high school days being "grossed out" at a football stadium upon seeing, a few rows away, a nursing mother. Disgusting! It was a shock, and in my adolescent mind I could not imagine why anyone would do such a thing.

Those traditional, learned attitudes fell by the wayside, however, when the time came for me actually to think about having my own baby. Once Rich and I felt we were ready, it took two-and-a-half years for me to get pregnant. I had more time than I wanted to observe our friends who were already there. By then, all my friends were nursing their newborns, and I knew that I would too. I wanted only the best for *my* child, and I was thoroughly convinced that breast milk was truly the best. When I fantasized becoming a mother, I was always cradling my dream child at my breast.

As is often the case, reality burst my bubble. After two miscarriages, one nearly fatal for me, we began to think of adoption. We endured two long, frustrating, and agonizing years of filling out forms, interviewing, more forms, checkups, and the interminable waiting required in adopting a child.

During that time came another pregnancy — this one a tubal pregnancy that ended abruptly when the tube burst and I was rushed to the emergency room, my veins collapsed, barely alive. The long recovery from abdominal surgery was sweetened only by the knowledge that our wait was almost over. Final approval from the adoption agency had come in the mail, and it was only a matter of time (how much, they would not say) until our dream would finally be realized. I could begin again to think about caring for my baby-to-be. My fantasy still included me holding my baby to my breast, but for a prospective adoptive mother, it seemed like an impossible dream.

Being a stubborn and determined person, I could not let go of the fantasy. I stumbled upon an article in a popular women's magazine about a mother who had breast-fed two biological children and then two adoptive children. Her situation was totally different from mine, but the seed of the idea was planted.

I called my doctor and asked if it were possible to nurse an adopted child. He said that it was possible in theory but not usually successful in practice — no encouragement there. I began to scour the libraries, searching for information on adoptive nursing. To my surprise, almost every book on nursing at least mentioned it. Tentatively encouraged, I called La Leche League and the leader I spoke to was friendly and helpful, but very cautious. She explained that it was difficult, time-consuming, and resulted in only varying degrees of success. This slight hint of encouragement was all I needed. I attended the next La Leche League meeting to get some information pamphlets on how to go about it. My determination was bolstered by the unbelievable support and encouragement these nursing women gave me. Until that meeting, everyone else, except my husband, had been skeptical, discouraging, even shocked, when I spoke about nursing an adopted baby. One pediatrician I called actually told me I was crazy. I hung up from that call and sobbed, filled with humiliation and anger. My emotional state was already very shaky from going through the adoption upheaval; it took very little to upset the balance. But finally I had found a group who did not question my motives, who could give me the emotional and technical support I needed.

I began to prepare in earnest for the difficult task I had set for myself. I ordered a device called a Lact-Aid, which is an aid to relactation and to induce lactation, invented by an adoptive couple. It was new to the market and seemed made just for my needs. It consists of a small plastic bag of formula, held in place by the mother's bra, from which comes a tiny, flexible tube that is placed on the nipple. As the baby nurses at the breast, he or she receives formula from the tube, and thus learns to expect milk from mother while at the same time stimulating the necessary hormones to begin their job of milk production. To use it I really needed my baby, but in the meantime I began toughening up my nipples and hand expressing milk. The results were meager, but my determination was undaunted. At least I was doing *something* while waiting. I found a pediatrician who was familiar with adoptive nursing and also encouraging. It meant driving across town, but that was a small price to pay for the moral support I received in return.

The long-awaited day finally came, and we were told to come and get our new son. To our surprise, Sean was six weeks old when he became ours and had been fed bottles and cereal by then. My spirits sagged: was it too late to make him a nurser? We had driven the two hundred miles to get him in a state of nervous anticipation and downright fear; as we brought him home we felt excited, frightened, and positively numb.

Rich went out immediately to buy forgotten necessities like diapers. Was I really prepared for this? I remained alone with my new son. He was fussy and fretful and I felt so stupid and helpless. As he fussed, my instinct told me to put him to my breast and to cuddle him. Even though I was completely alone at the time, I felt ridiculous. I hadn't even bought the Lact-Aid yet because I thought the excitement would be too great for all of us. So there I was, finally a mother, with an unhappy, fretful child in my arms. I put him to my breast, and he immediately settled down. Tears streaming down my face, I rocked my little son to sleep, and my fantasy was finally fulfilled.

We established a new mother/new baby routine, and I gradually switched from mostly bottle feedings to mostly Lact-Aid feedings. In nine days I was able to express drops of breast milk. By the three-month checkup, the doctor estimated that I was providing ten ounces of milk a day. Sean decided that his mother was not supposed to use a bottle at all and would not take one from me, although he would from his father or a sitter.

I spent practically all of my time learning about this new child of mine. We established the close bond that nursing couples often do, and we carry this with us even six years later. I chose literally to devote myself to nursing this adopted child, and I have never regretted it for one instant. He needs me less each day now, but those months we spent in such close contact will remain with us forever. My fantasy of motherhood has undergone many changes as reality has taught me one lesson after another over the years. But I was able to do something that I wanted and needed desperately: nurse my adopted child.

———————

Three years later, I gave birth to a little girl, three months prematurely. At two-pounds-one-and-a-half ounces, Marisa needed every "extra" benefit I could give her. I had stayed flat on my back for four-and-a-half months during my pregnancy, trying to carry her to term. I had also insisted on going through the delivery without any kind of medication to give the baby every possible chance. When she finally came home from the hospital at seven weeks of age, weighing all of four pounds, my experience of nursing Sean made it much easier to nurse his little sister. I used the same techniques to build up a milk supply and nursed her even in the special care nursery. I told Sean how I had nursed him when he was a baby; we both felt happy about it.

Things have progressed a great deal since I nursed my adopted child. More doctors today are willing to help adoptive mothers begin building up a milk supply even before they get their babies. The Lact-Aid is still the major help to relactating women. More people today have heard about adoptive nursing and are not nearly as surprised, or horrified, as they were then. However, I still run across people — even medical people — who are unknowledgeable about it.

I am glad that I followed my instincts and persevered to get what I wanted and needed for myself and for my children.

GLORIA BENNETT plans to return to teaching or find a new career. "After working so hard to achieve it, I believe that motherhood is worth a one-hundred-percent effort," she says. "For now, by wiping noses and reading stories I am doing the most important job for myself and my family." The Bennetts live in Garland, Texas.

A Letter from a Natural Mother

DEBORAH FERRIS BRYAN

Dear Son,

I was fifteen years old and unmarried when I learned that I was pregnant with you. I had to decide very quickly what to do.

The boy who had fathered you decided that it was love only until he got caught.

I had the choice of keeping you or turning over your care and upbringing to a couple who could guide and nurture you. I gave you up not because I didn't love or want you, but because I was smart enough to know that I would be unable to give you all the attention, love, and support that you would need to make it through the rough times in life. I hoped that the couple who would open their hearts and door to you would have the patience, love, and maturity that I was lacking as a teenager.

I was allowed to hold you one time, and when the nurse handed you to me I could imagine the day when she would be handing you to the woman soon to become your mother. When the time came to sign the final adoption papers, I did so with tears in my eyes and a longing in my heart. Yet I knew that your parents were going to be shedding tears too, tears of joy and thankfulness for their new-found son.

There are so many questions inside of me concerning you, my son. I wonder if you made it through infancy, and whether you had teething problems or diaper rash. I wonder how old you were when you took your first step. Did you learn to use the potty easily, or did it cause your mother early graying? I wonder if when you went to school for the first time, you had tears in your eyes and a smile on your face. Are you shy and retiring, or bold and brassy?

I also wonder if you ever ask about me. Have you ever been told that you are adopted? Do you wonder about your natural father? Do you understand my reasons for giving you up? I was not ready to accept the responsibility of guiding your life before I was capable of guiding my own. By giving you up to this couple, who I felt had so much more to offer you than I had, I hope that I gave you the freedom to live, to love, and to learn with two parents who truly want you.

Do you know that now, only nine years later, people consider what I did, giving you up, to be appalling and disgusting? How could anyone give up their own flesh and blood? they ask. But they cannot fully comprehend what conflicts arise inside a young girl faced with the dilemma of raising an infant alone. I know that I made the right decision, and I hope that you will understand that it was my love for you that guided me.

264

My son, on your birthday my heart opens up and searches the world, trying to discover where and how you are. Are you happy? Do you look back on each year with pride and forward to the coming year with a feeling of joy and a desire to make it better than the last one?

I sometimes wonder what the people who are close to me would think if they knew that I have a son who is living his life with someone else. My husband can't bring himself to let me tell him about the feelings I have for you, but he does try not to disturb or disrupt those feelings.

Perhaps someday we shall meet; that will have to be your decision. Until then, my love and prayers are with you every day of my life.

> Lovingly,
> Your Natural Mother

DEBORAH FERRIS BRYAN and her husband, David, have four children. The oldest was born when she was sixteen and not yet married. "When we did marry, eleven months after his birth, we knew that it was not because we 'had to,' but because we wanted to and because we loved each other." Deborah, a secretary for her local hospital's Pediatric Guild, lives in Hastings, Michigan.

16

Teenage Mothers

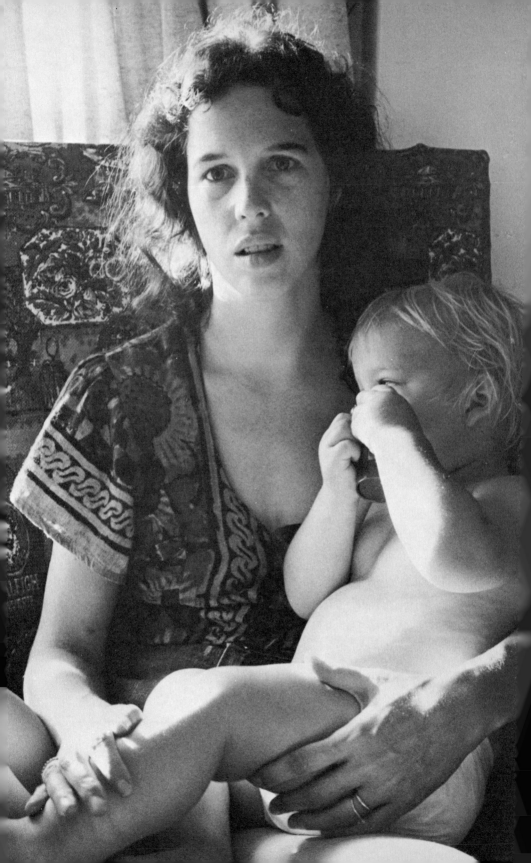

Motherhood at Sixteen

DANA GILBERT

The frightening story that we all heard and never believed became a living reality: the first time I ever made love, I became pregnant. And it had actually happened to me, the sixteen-year-old know-it-all who supposedly understood all about sex.

When I found out for certain, I kept thinking to myself, I didn't do enough to get pregnant. There has to be more to getting pregnant than that. It must be a mistake.

My life began to flash before me so fast, I couldn't even think straight. Fragments passed in and out of my mind — boyfriend, family, school, friends, my future — what was I going to do? I wanted to scream as loud as I could and cry forever, but I held myself together and called my boyfriend at work. He is a construction worker and wasn't near a telephone. I had to wait for someone to locate him and for him to call me back. That was the longest and loneliest time I've ever spent.

I tried to think of a clever way to tell him that, at the ripe old age of nineteen, he was going to become a father. Finally the phone rang. I blurted out the news. Much to my amazement, he took it very calmly and was actually pleased.

That afternoon we got together and planned the next step — our marriage. I know it sounds like the classic story of two people who made a mistake and were getting married to correct it. But in spite of our youth, we loved each other deeply.

We decided to get married about a month from the day I found out I was expecting. I would finish the tenth grade of high school before marrying and becoming a mother.

My first day back at school after discovering my pregnancy was memorable. I told all my friends that I was to be married in a month, deliberately neglecting to tell them about being pregnant.

Of course they were shocked. Although no one asked me directly, I'm sure they were wondering why so soon.

Before that day was over, I saw my friends in a different light. They all seemed so babyish looking and silly, giggling and laughing about everything. They didn't seem to have a care in the world.

I began to withdraw from them, not because I wanted to, but because we had nothing in common anymore. I wasn't interested in flirting with David or Ricky, or concerned with what kind of bikini I was going to get for the summer. I became a loner with only one close friend with whom I could talk.

As the weeks went by and my wedding day came and went, some of my schoolmates realized that I was pregnant. I remember one friend told me that she was sorry but she could no longer be friends with me or even talk to me. When I asked her why, she said her mother didn't want her hanging around with a girl of my "kind." I denied being pregnant to her and to everyone else who even hinted at it. After all, I didn't have a contagious disease; I was still the same me I'd always been; I'd just had to grow up a little faster than the other girls.

Soon the pregnancy began to show physically. One day in English class my baby moved for the first time. I was so excited that I wanted to shout, "Hey, my baby's kicking; it's really kicking." Yet I couldn't tell anyone except my one close friend. I couldn't pay any attention in class that day, or the many that followed. The school year finally ended, and I thought I had lived through the hardest part of my pregnancy — having had to deny it to my classmates. By this time there was no more denying it.

That summer and fall, everywhere I went, whether it was just buying groceries or shopping, I heard whispers and received nasty stares.

Funny, to most of them I was no longer Dana, a nice little girl; I was someone who had turned "bad." They made me feel ashamed and dirty. I shouldn't have let their negative feelings bother me so, but they did.

The days slowly crept by, and on a fall day I gave birth to a beautiful girl. All the monstrous remarks that had made me feel guilty for months seemed meaningless once she was born.

DANA GILBERT is a pseudonym.

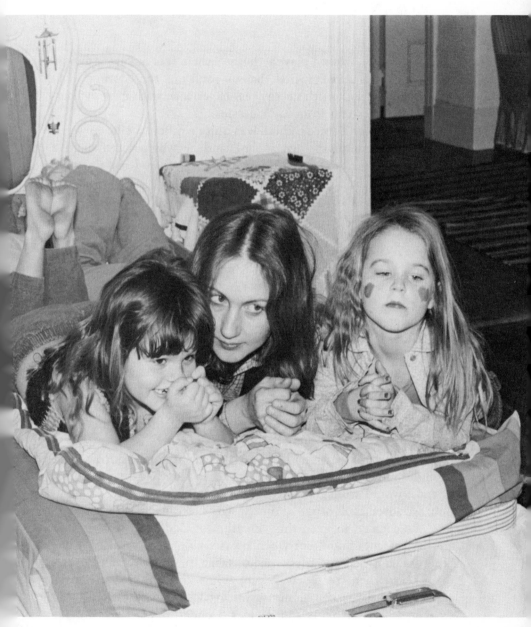

Joan Albert

A Teenager's Point of View

SUSAN A. ROTH

Like other girls, when I played "house" there was always a loving, gentle husband; a sweet, little baby — and me, the adoring, loyal wife. Little did I expect that my real experience with new motherhood would be so far from my fantasies.

When I met Tommy, there was quite a difference in our ages. I was a sophomore in high school, and he was a foreman in a construction company. It was wonderful — just as I had dreamed — bells ringing and colorful fireworks.

I matured greatly the first half-year that I was seeing him. Other girls were going to dances, cheerleading, and doing things that seemed suddenly childish to me.

We had a difficult time because of the strictness of both of our families. He couldn't come to the house; I had to say that I was going to a friend's home and meet him secretly. Looking back on it, all the intrigue helped romanticize my feelings for him even more.

When school was finally over, my life with Tommy began. We had a beautiful summer romance, spending every glorious day together. But then the nightmare started. Autumn came. The leaves had turned from a cool green to a crisp brown. I never thought it would happen, but it did. I became pregnant. At first I was happy. I had just turned seventeen. Was I ready to become a mother? Yes, I was. I loved Tommy, and I would love our baby just as much.

But Tommy wasn't too pleased when he found out and immediately decided on an abortion. For three months I fought against it, and I won. I wondered why he had wanted me to have an abortion: we loved each other so much; why destroy a part of us?

We decided to keep this "creation of God" and work things out. My parents found out when I was six months pregnant. I had been too confused and frightened of what they would think to tell them before then. Yet I was so happy! Just knowing that there was a little part of me and Tommy waiting to be born thrilled me. I crocheted little blankets and bootees, wondering whether to make them pink or blue.

272

A week before the wedding, Tommy left the country. My dreams all vanished with him. I was terribly hurt and shocked. It was the worst time in my life. I knew I had some serious decisions to make. But I had fought for this baby in the beginning, and I was not going to abandon it just because the father had left me.

My parents, however, decided differently. They said that if I kept the baby, I would not be allowed back in the house. They wanted me to go to a home for unwed mothers. I was totally opposed to that. My decision had already been made: I was going to keep my baby whether I could bring her home or not. So I went to social services to see if they could get me an apartment until I got back on my feet. I was praying they would say yes, but they informed me that I wasn't of legal age and my parents were still responsible.

I thought I was going to go crazy. Things were so bad that I attempted to base my decision on fate: if I had a boy, I knew that it was meant for me to give it up; but if I had a girl, I knew that it was meant for me to keep it.

All I felt at that time was deep anger. Why was everyone trying to hurt me? I was in a daze for weeks, unable to think. Why couldn't I be happy like other mothers-to-be? I felt I was being cheated of a very special time. Then, a week before my baby was due, my parents said that I could bring the baby home. A feeling of peace such as I have never before experienced came over me. Finally I could start putting my life together.

On Father's Day, ironically, Taralyn Marie, a girl, of course, was born. She was the picture of perfection, my little bundle of joy. She was the only one who had stuck by me in my despair.

Being in the hospital was difficult for me. The woman in the next bed had her husband with her all the time, bringing her presents and acting proud. How I wanted Tommy to be with us.

It took me a while to get used to taking care of Taralyn, but with my two brothers, sister, and wonderful mother and father (I realize now that they were doing what they thought would have been the best for me) she always has a lot of love and attention. I hope she gets enough to make up for her father not being there. My own father changed from "I won't even look at her" to having her become the apple of Grandpa's eye. I never felt such love in our house before. I believe that this baby is here for the purpose of bringing us all closer together as a family.

At first everybody acted sort of strange; we were all brought up thinking pregnancy before marriage is taboo. But they soon realized that things are different today, and that my baby was conceived out of a deep love.

Although I adore taking care of my daughter and observing her grow day by day, I watched all my friends going out to discos and such, and I felt cheated by having to stay home and take care of her. I missed a very important part of my life. I grew up too fast. I still want to go out, but my daughter comes first, and she always will. I love her very much and wouldn't go back on my decision for anything.

I think there is a motherly instinct in every woman. It's like a sixth sense, knowing Taralyn's wants and needs, and knowing that she is completely dependent upon me. It is the most beautiful feeling I have ever experienced in my whole life. We're going to have a very special life; I'm going to see to it.

A while ago, when Taralyn was eight months old, Tommy called. I was both excited and upset. Why was he trying to disrupt our lives when I was just pulling everything together? I agreed to see him because I would like my daughter to know her father, for him to hold her, and for just one time to have the feeling that we are a family. In some ways, I would still like to have a "dream house" with a white picket fence.

Tommy and I may get together someday, but only if I feel the trust I once had in him, and only if I believe that my daughter would benefit from his presence. She will never be hurt by him as I was. Next time, I will not let childish emotions get the better of me.

SUSAN ROTH is eighteen and lives in West Babylon, New York, with her father, an electrician, and her mother, who works in a nursing home. "I am trying to finish beauty school and to make a life for myself and for my daughter."

17

Feelings About Surgical Deliveries

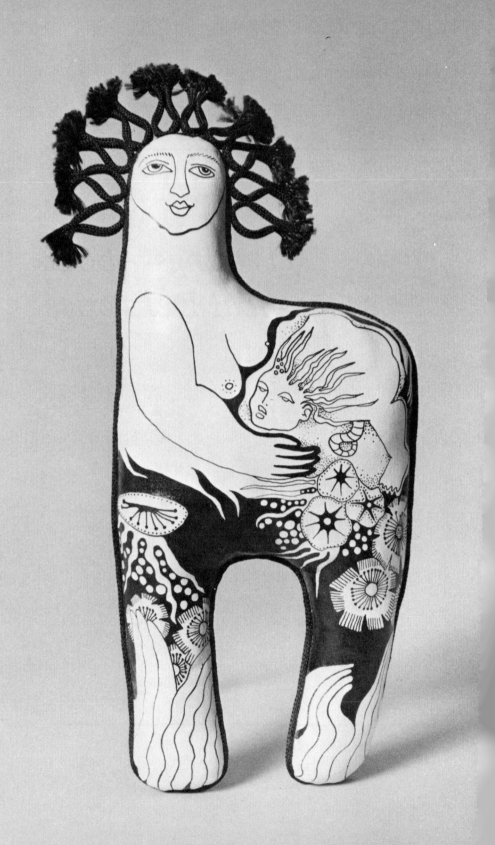

Birth/Caesarean

CAROL HOFFMAN DeCANIO

At night
under one light
a woman scrapes a razor across my humped
    stomach
and tears through all that is hidden

She asks the names of my children
I play her game
as she inspects my body
a white fish fillet

A man comes in
talking of numbness
tomorrow is the day
I choose from his plate

While alone with the ceiling
another knocks
the pill patrol
enforcing sleep
I say no

In the morning
nothing by mouth

A woman comes in
I do what she says
curl tight on my side
cling to the bars
as a plastic tube winds
into my rectum
and soap suds jerk
at the bowel

I sit on the toilet
and read a mystery

As I again find the bed
two women arrive with a needle
they shoot good feelings
into my hip

The enema woman returns
with her new invention
a tube to get my urine
and I lay open.
She pushes it in slowly
and I watch a plastic purse
turn yellow.
I wear it.
She sees my wedding band
calculates
I can wear it
after it's taped to my finger

The door opens differently
two men wheel in a plank
it rushes my bed
Slide Over
a surgical cap
is whipped on my head
lopsided

We whoosh out the door
we stop at the desk
everyone seems to be standing
talking of another world
my lips press tight
the nurse touches my cheek

I close my eyes against the standing world
and open them on the first floor
before the flapping doors
of the operating room

I wait in the hall
a man stands beside me
reading papers
talking of numbness
as we enter the room.
It gleams.

I stare back at the round flat light
as a needle trailing tubes
is pushed in my arm.
Don't Move
a tube of promises
is shot into my spine
Don't Move

Across my chest
vertical metal
clicks into place
flung with sheets, sheets

My stomach is pricked
Done?
And I don't even feel the first slice

Hands push down hard
again, again
something shoves out
gurgles, small cries

You have a fine boy, he says
A woman brings him to me in a wrapper
and I touch his cheek

Caesarean — Not the Right Way

PAULA ROACH WHEELER

"Your baby is breech. There is a possibility that you may have to have a Caesarean." These words, spoken by the resident after we arrived at the hospital for the birth of our first child, had little effect on me. Surely our baby would turn, and I would be able to deliver naturally; surely our Lamaze classes would not be in vain. Caesareans happened to *other* women.

After I spent three hours in the last stages of labor, however, our doctor made the decision: surgery. Exhausted, I was relieved to know the contractions, which had produced nothing but pain, would soon end. I was also relieved not to have to imagine the urge to push, which I never felt. Our baby would be born, and it would all be over.

There was no way to gauge the amount of time that elapsed during the endless ride to surgery, the swabbing and prepping of my aching stomach, the IVs. My husband, my source of emotional support, was left behind. I felt frantic when my arms and legs were secured, taking away even more of my ability to participate. The large plastic mask, which was supposed to be anchored over my nose and mouth, refused to stay in place.

I saw no faces. I was surrounded by sterile chrome and moving figures in white and green. I concentrated as best I could on my breathing, my last bit of control, trying also to tell myself that once the decision was made for surgery, it must be carried out as expeditiously as possible. I remember thinking: I must cooperate, I must be brave, I must not panic. I was trying to cooperate, I was trying to be brave, but I was also panicking. I wanted to hear from my doctor, whom I trusted, to have him tell me that things would be all right.

Finally, a moment before the green cloth separated my torso from the rest of my body, I saw my doctor. I felt a glimmer of hope, a moment of reassurance. But then irrational fear took over: would he know that I was still awake, still experiencing the endless contractions, still fighting the oxygen mask? What if he began before I was asleep? These were my last, nightmarish thoughts before surrendering to the anesthetic.

I awoke in the recovery room, extremely confused. My husband told me that we had a healthy, red-headed baby boy. He had seen the baby in the nursery, and our son was fine. Despite its casualness, "Gee, that's nice" seemed sufficient as I drifted back to sleep.

On my ride from recovery to my room, through the nursery window, my husband and I saw a bundle of blankets, topped by a beautiful red head. So that was our baby . . .

Twelve hours after his birth, my head had cleared enough to want to see him for myself. With a great deal of difficulty, and much encouragement and assistance from the nurses, I was able to hold him and nurse him. But the nurses had to change him from one side to the other, and I was aggravated at my limpness and at the tubes which got in the way. I was amazed at his smallness and at the softness of his head and skin. Then he was taken away, and again I slept; this soon became my routine.

Although our family, our friends, and everyone else seemed thrilled and excited, I, the mother, really did not feel these emotions for quite some time. I was certainly pleased with our son, but in no way did I feel I was a part of the events. Perhaps it was the loss of half a day with no recollections, while the effects of the anesthetic wore off. The memory of my surgery was fresh in my mind. The pain in my abdomen grew with every movement I made, and I dreaded the thought of looking at the incision. I didn't feel like a person — I was a thing, a groggy nonentity stuck full of needles, attached to tubes, and encircled by hanging bottles.

The next day the IVs came out and the needles and tubes were withdrawn. I finally was allowed some ice chips, a treat for which I had yearned from the time I entered the labor room but which had been forbidden fruit. The ecstasy of the ice chips, however, was quickly replaced by the agony of my twenty-five-minute adventure to the bathroom, located in my room. As I inched my way along, each movement was a great effort — I feared I'd never make it. Easing back into bed with the speed of a snail drove home all the harder the fact that I had indeed given birth the hard way.

After the first day, our son was brought in at regular intervals for his meals, and I soon grew to look forward to these moments to hold, touch, sing, or talk to him. His visits were a peaceful time, a soothing balm to my troubled mind. Just watching him I could feel my tensions melting away.

But there was still a flaw for me in the excitement. Although he looked like his father and he had my hair color, in some strange way I didn't *feel* he was mine. I remember thinking that perhaps this was how a father might have felt in the days when he could not be present for his child's birth. It was as though I too had not been there, as though it had never happened. There was a void in my life, a period beyond recollection. Something that had been a part of me for so long had suddenly materialized, as if by magic, as a new little person.

As the days wore on in the hospital, and some of my mobility returned, Chad became more familiar to me, and I became more involved with him. Nonetheless, whenever I shuffled down to the nursery with family or friends, I shared their amazement at seeing our son. I kept feeling that I too was seeing him for the first time.

On the fifth day my stitches were taken out. I became brave enough to look at my scar and hoped the doctors and nurses were right when they said I would not pop open if I laughed or coughed. It just felt that way.

At the end of my week in the hospital, I was able to nurse Chad unassisted. It was a herky-jerky process, but he did not break and was quite patient with my efforts. My confidence finally took one giant step forward.

————————

Coming home was an attractive idea, but the reality of caring for a baby when I could barely walk, much less bend and stoop, was not. I feared failing at home, as I felt I had in the labor room.

For the first two weeks at home, my husband seemed to be everywhere, doing everything that the hospital staff had done. What he could not do, unfortunately, was take my mind off the trauma of our son's birth. It stayed with me long after I was able to concentrate on caring for our baby boy. When I attempted any menial chores while Chad slept, my mind would slowly return to the events of his birth. The scar and soreness were constant reminders.

My goal toward the end of pregnancy had been small enough — I simply wanted to sleep on my stomach. Now even this was denied me. During the pregnancy I had felt helpless and longed for the birth to be over so that I could again control my body. Now, it was not happening; instead, my body was still dictating to me. Trying to rise from a chair while holding the baby, getting into or out of bed, or changing the crib sheets were small activities but continual hurdles, given my slow recovery.

After my husband returned to work, he still would help whenever and wherever he could. He was patient with my curtness and loving throughout the tears; but my anger was there, my frustration was building. The omnipresent question was: Why do I have to do things the difficult way? We had lost an earlier pregnancy and this one had been less than picture perfect, with spotting and intermittent bleeding, bedrest, and confinement for two months. Why couldn't I do something right for a change?

My discouragement created a vicious circle, one that was hard to break. On the surface, we appeared to have an ideal situation: our son was healthy and happy; I was nursing him; and Dad had things under control. It was the perfect family setting. In reality, though, I was struggling through the days, unable to get out of the house, unable to drive, feeling punk for six weeks. For me these were all radical changes. Before I became pregnant I was always on the go, with one or two projects in progress. I could be packed in twenty minutes for a week-long trip. I thrived on people and on both serious and frivolous conversations.

After our son's birth, however, just as during the middle two months of my pregnancy, I was confined to quarters, my mobility limited and my mind preoccupied with personal thoughts. I could not explain why I could not cope with my new situation, why my attitude deteriorated so dramatically. To all outward appearances I was the independent, self-sufficient person I had always been.

My husband and I, however, were aware that my enormous attitudinal changes presented a grave problem. My erratic moods, my lack of any positive outlook, and my absence of enthusiasm caused a great deal of strain between us. Reestablishing a physical relationship was particularly difficult. Intellectually my husband's needs were easy to understand, but emotionally I found a barrier of fear and resentment when it came to physical affection.

As with all new mothers, first and foremost I was tired. Not getting my usual amount of sleep was a problem in itself. On top of that I was preoccupied, distracted, and unable to relax because of the operation. With the surgery on my mind, it was hard to disassociate lovemaking from pregnancy. And I dreaded becoming pregnant again.

My mental recuperation received a substantial boost when Chad was two months old. I became involved in a project with friends that got me out of the house each night for two weeks. And then a friend and I collaborated to enable me to hold a part-time afternoon job. She watched Chad while I worked, and we split the earnings. It was good for all of us, particularly me. At the same time, I joined a bowling league. As I began to resume outside activities, I found I had much less time to be depressed.

───────────

Just as I was picking up the pieces and putting things in proper perspective, my worst apprehensions were realized: despite my precautions, I was pregnant again, only fourteen months after the first birth.

I was back at square one, and for the next eight months I experienced the same anxieties I had hoped were gone. I considered requesting a spinal anesthetic for the surgery I dreaded, so that I could be aware of the birth of our second child. I tried to prepare mentally, telling myself that this time I would have an idea of what to expect. At least this time I would not be so exhausted from the hours of futile labor.

In the end, my fears proved needless. As a result of unexpected and happy circumstances, I was able to deliver our daughter vaginally.

That was almost a year ago. My fears — both physical and emotional — have finally faded away. I wish I could share the magic formula that helped me to regain my previous positive outlook, but I'm not sure there was one.

I know that Rachel's normal birth, which was as unscheduled as the Caesarean had been, played a large part in my psychological recovery. Add to this the joy of participating in Chad's growth into a loving, happy little boy who was thrilled by his new sister. Finally,

I suppose time — the proverbial healer — did its share. Now the whole experience is a far-off memory.

Although many of my reactions could have been anticipated, at the time it was as if no one else had gone through a Caesarean. As any new mother can attest, there are days when you believe that no one can appreciate the emotions you are experiencing, that no one has been where you are. I hope that I can help other mothers, beset by some of these same anxieties, to realize that they are not alone in their feelings of confusion and isolation.

PAULA ROACH WHEELER was twenty-nine and working as a children's librarian in Springfield, Illinois, when her son was born. She plans to wait until her children are in school before resuming her career.

Caesarean — Not the Wrong Way

CATHY HEENAN

Two weeks before my due date, my doctor offered a seminar for all the couples who expected to have a child that month. There were seven couples in the room. The doctor looked at us and said, "One of you seven women will have a Caesarean." I glanced around the room and whispered to my husband, "I wonder which one of *them* it will be."

That night, at two in the morning, two weeks early, my water broke, and I went into labor. I had arranged for a midwife to be present at my child's birth. Janet arrived at my home in the early morning and examined me. I was one centimeter dilated and almost completed effaced. Janet monitored my contractions, and at noon, when they were five minutes apart, we all left for the hospital.

Two hours later, my labor became quite hard; the contractions were coming every three to four minutes apart, and the only way I could manage the pain was by standing up, leaning on my husband Bob, and swaying. All of us assumed that the labor was progressing well.

But when my doctor, John, examined me, I was only two centimeters dilated. In the early evening he returned to examine me again. Still, I was only two centimeters dilated: virtually no change for seven-and-a-half hours! I had been working terribly hard, and nothing had happened. I was upset, frustrated, confused, and beginning to panic. What was wrong? Why wasn't I opening? Such work and pain for nothing. Why wasn't I moving any closer to delivering my baby?

John determined that Pitocin would not be used (I was not dilating, but my contractions were strong). I continued to labor, with contractions coming every three minutes. With enormous hope, I lay on the table as John again examined me. His eyes told me all: no change. As I heard his words, I burst into tears. I was frightened, vulnerable, and filled with enormous loss. He began to talk of a Caesarean section. It was as if I had never heard the words before. What would it mean for me to have a Caesarean? What effect would it have on the baby? Might I die? What kind of medication would I have? What effect would the medication have on the baby? What about my husband's participation in the birth experience? How would I bond with my child? Could I nurse? And how in the world could I take care of my baby while recovering from an operation? With each question, I became increasingly anxious.

All my plans and dreams for a gentle birth suddenly vanished. I looked at Bob, longing for him to have some magical answer. I saw the pain and sadness in his eyes. I looked at Janet and asked her if she agreed with John. Did I really need a Caesarean? She answered yes. I wept, and so did Bob. In desperation, I asked what would happen if I kept on with the labor; what were the odds that I would dilate fully? The answer was, barely a chance. Nothing indicated that there would be any change a few hours from now. Janet and John left the room. Bob and I talked, we cried, and we decided to have the Caesarean. I didn't want to continue with the labor any longer. There seemed no point in trying to manage the pain, which was not creating what needed to be created — a large enough opening through which the baby could pass. All I wanted by that point was for my baby to be delivered safely.

———

Hospital technicians began to arrive, as well as hospital administrators. I felt intruded upon to have these people asking me questions. What type of medication would I like? Do I want to be awake or asleep? I barely remember the questions, yet I can still see the outline of the unfamiliar faces looming around me.

Bob, Janet, and John were wonderful advocates, and I sorely needed advocates. Each time I had a contraction, John asked the administrators and technicians to step back so he could work with me during the contraction. He never forgot me. He never forgot that my feelings were important. He made others wait for me. He did not make me wait. He assured me that Bob would be with me, and that he would be as gentle and as loving as possible with the baby. And he assured me that although we would be in an operating room, we could and would have a loving birth. I believed him; I needed to. And he was telling the truth.

During the last few contractions, before I was given the spinal, I kept seeing rows and rows of red tulips. I told John this, and as I was given the spinal, he talked to me and told me to see those tulips, "the yellow ones, the red ones, and the orange ones." In my madness, I said to him, "No, there are only red tulips." He helped me see the tulips. He was in touch with my experience and responsive to me. And the spinal did not hurt.

As I lay on the operating table waiting for surgery, I talked to every person in the delivery room: the head nurse, the anesthesiologist, the doctor assisting my doctor, the pediatrician, and the technicians. I told them what we had hoped for in a birthing room, and asked them to be gentle. They were. The anesthesiologist, who had been cold to me an hour before as he routinely asked me whether I wanted to be put to sleep or stay awake, was now rubbing my forehead and assuring me that all would be fine. The pediatrician assured me that he would examine the baby gently, and the head nurse smiled encouragingly.

My arms shook and my teeth chattered as I lay on the cold operating table. A screen was placed in front of me so I could not see. The lower half of my body was deadened. It was so awful and paradoxical to feel nothing after nineteen hours of feeling so much. Bob was sitting beside me dressed in hospital attire and masked. He touched me and talked to me. Thank goodness he was with me. I was uncomfortable, but able to feel the kindness of the people, and to hear the quietness of the room.

Then I heard John say, "We're going to begin now." I felt tugging and pulling, stretching and pressure. I was very uncomfortable. I told him this, and Janet whispered, "It is better not to have any additional medication since you want to nurse." I clenched Bob's hand more tightly. Minutes seemed like an eternity. I kept wishing my teeth would stop chattering and my jaw would stop aching. Then John saw the baby. A little more stretching and pulling, and I heard him exclaim, "I've got the baby. Your baby is a girl." And I remember saying, "It's a girl. It's a girl. Oh, Babe, we have a girl."

Tears streamed down my face, and I was flooded with joy and relief. The pediatrician quickly examined her. The baby was crying. He handed her to Bob, then whispered to me, "She's perfect." Bob removed his mask, opened his gown, and held her to his breast. She stopped crying. Not a sound. He held her in his arms next to his heart, and they looked at one another. I held her little foot. We both talked quietly to our daughter.

They both stayed with me for a while, and then Bob took our daughter to the recovery room and turned off all the lights, so she could more fully open her eyes. They sat together bonding with one another. Janet stayed with me. Once I knew that the baby was safe and with her papa, I experienced my own pain more deeply. Janet had me breathe as if I were still in labor. I kept asking John, "How much longer until it's over?" It was as if I were five years old, riding in my father's car and saying, "When are we going to get there, Daddy?" John kept saying, "Only a few minutes more." I watched the clock. It took more than a few minutes to close me up — more like thirty minutes. I was hurting badly. And then it was over. I was being wheeled into the recovery room to join Bob and my baby. Bob looked transformed. He was so excited and filled with love as he placed our daughter beside me. She turned her head toward my breast and nursed easily. Bob and I touched as our daughter nursed. Finally, we were alone. The three of us.

—————

Yes, we delivered our daughter in an operating room. Yes, a Caesarean section is major surgery. Yes, I could not hold her immediately after her birth. And yes, I was enormously disappointed not to have gone through natural childbirth. Yet, despite all of this, I learned a lot. I learned that birth by Caesarean can be gentle and loving. I learned that my husband could participate in our surgical birth and that he could bond with our baby; and that I could join them both shortly afterward and nurse without difficulty. I learned the importance and necessity of good, humanized medical care. I learned, once again, how essential it is to trust those who will help you make significant decisions. I learned that my body has limits over which I have no control. I learned that the kind of birth I wanted was insignificant in comparison to my desire to have a healthy baby. For me, there could be no ego in having a child. I learned that what I expect and hope for doesn't always happen, and that I can survive and even benefit from the unexpected, as well as from disappointments.

All the fears during my pregnancy faded as I gazed at my daughter's beautiful face and held her warm little body in my arms. I was grateful that she was fine, and that I was fine. I felt blessed.

CATHY HEENAN became a mother when she was thirty-three. She returned to work part time as a psychotherapist and human relations consultant in the Boston area when her daughter was two months old. Cathy has also co-authored a book and worked on her dissertation.

Premature Birth and the Aftermath

DALE FRIEDLAND DANIELS

My introduction to motherhood was nothing like the natural childbirth I had hoped for and expected. I did not have a normal labor and delivery. In the thirty-third week of my pregnancy, I had an emergency Caesarean section; my total labor consisted of two contractions that I saw on a monitor, but hardly felt. My own life was at stake, and for two very long weeks, my baby's survival was questioned. Eventually we both were healed physically, but for me the emotional healing process has taken much longer.

The first indication that my pregnancy was going awry was when I began spotting. I was examined and had a sonagram, which indicated that my child appeared healthy, my placenta intact, and my cervix closed. Nevertheless, after several hours of vague discomfort, a decision was made to monitor me throughout the night. The assumption was that I would leave the hospital in the morning.

For the first few hours everything was fine. Then we noticed a contraction on the monitor. From that point on, things happened so quickly that within two hours the decision was made for me to have a Caesarean section. I do not clearly remember the actual sequence of events, but I will never forget the intensity of the feelings accompanying them.

I was immediately given a vasodilator to stop the contractions. This resulted in nausea, dizziness, and ultimately drowsiness. I struggled to stay awake and absorb what was going on around me, knowing that it was the only way I could retain some semblance of control over the situation. But I was frustrated by my sleepiness and embarrassed and frightened by my body's behavior. I apologized for vomiting and for my inability to take care of my basic physical needs.

I accepted with ease their decision to do a Caesarean section. I heard all the facts: my placenta was abrupting, and although there was not yet any sign of fetal distress, they needed to go ahead and deliver my baby. The danger to me was the hemorrhaging into my uterus between the placenta and the uterine wall. I felt in control again when I signed my medical release, opted for spinal anesthesia, and learned that my husband could stay with me in surgery. That helped a great deal. Steven would be there for me. I knew I could rely on him, and so I felt safe.

It was when they were wheeling me down the hall to surgery that I learned the situation had changed. Because it was a complicated delivery (transverse fetal lie), I needed to be put under general anesthesia, and Steven could not be present. I panicked. Suddenly

I felt terrified that I was going to die. I prayed repeatedly. I was so afraid I was dying that when they told me they were going to put me out, I silently recited the Shema, the last words a Jew is supposed to say before death.

When I awoke, and throughout the next few days, I tried to obliterate from my mind the fact that my life had been threatened. I blocked out most of the events of the night, remembering the sense of fear but not its cause. I pushed to get my body functioning normally as soon as possible in order to feel in control again. The speed at which I became ambulatory was almost a medical miracle. Nevertheless, I considered my body a traitor: it had failed me. It was difficult to accept that no cause could be found for what had happened. My family and I carefully reviewed my activities, and the fact that we couldn't come up with a particular incident to blame relieved everyone's guilt but no one's anxiety. It would have been easier to accept the consequences if there had been a reason.

As soon as the immediate fear for my own survival had passed, my concern was for my son, Aaron. He was born seven weeks prematurely, and it was obvious from his initial exam that all was not well. His weight was good, but his color indicated respiratory distress. Within a few hours, he developed hyaline membrane disease, a condition resulting from prematurity in which breathing is inadequate. He was placed on a respirator, his condition was poor, and the first seventy-two hours would be critical.

I first saw Aaron about nine hours after his birth. They wheeled me on a stretcher, and I looked through the window of the Intensive Care Nursery (ICN). I could hardly see his face because of the respirator, but I could see his hair and his tiny naked body. It's a sight I still remember as clearly as if it just happened — so different from how I had first planned to see my baby. I tried to associate the little boy behind the glass with the life I had felt in my womb, but I felt distant. I remember saying that I thought he looked like one of my nephews. He didn't, but I needed some tangible association with him.

The contrast between my situation and what I had hoped for was underscored when I later arrived at my room. The impersonal organization of a hospital can be terribly cruel. I had been placed in a room with a mother who had elected to have her healthy child room in with her. At first their presence was not too difficult. But as time passed, the cooing and feeding sounds became increasingly painful. Fortunately, upon the urging of my family, a sensitive nurse arranged to switch me to a private room.

It was that same day that I finally felt close to my son. I couldn't hold him; I could hardly see him; but I was able to reach up and touch his legs. I sat there afraid to leave, afraid that I might never see him alive again. That fear haunted me for the next several days.

———————

The third day was a nightmare. My husband had to return to work. My parents had returned to their home. I was alone. When I got to the ICN, a new resident met me with upsetting news about Aaron. The baby had suffered through a very bad night. They feared he had a congenital heart problem.

I remember the noise and bustle of the ICN. I remember the way the resident smiled as she told me this latest piece of news. And I remember looking at Aaron and starting to cry. They were the first tears that I had shed since I had arrived at the hospital. And with those tears began a grieving for what had happened to me, and for what was happening to my baby. Throughout that day the intensity of my sadness grew. Friends visited and saw Aaron through the ICN window. Their shock at his condition was torturous for me, but further shook me out of the numbness I had been experiencing the past few days. Now I hurt badly, but it was good to be finally feeling again. The sadness was almost overwhelming. But for the first time, I believed Aaron would survive. I began to let myself experience all my pain and disappointment. I questioned why I had failed to carry my child to term — my inability to nurture and protect my child made me feel inadequate as a mother. I wondered what aftereffects the experience might have on Aaron. Could I cope with problems should they arise? It was the beginning of questioning and understanding myself as a mother.

Throughout this difficult period and through the next few months, my relationships with others affected my feelings. My husband was my support, at times giving me the will to continue to live. From the moment the trauma began, he was honest with me about everything. He was so devastated, yet so sensitive. The pain of the experience was lessened by the closeness we shared.

My immediate family was there for me too. Their support was immeasurable. Yet even with them I masked my feelings about the situation. To let go totally, I felt, would have made me their child. I couldn't be that when I needed to be Aaron's mother.

So many others also cared and helped immeasurably. It seemed as if everyone who knew us prayed with us. A well-meaning few offered us platitudes that all would be well. How I wanted to strangle them! I wanted prayers, not platitudes.

With each day that passed, there were new ups and downs. At five days, Aaron was removed from the respirator. I finally held my baby. Shortly thereafter, I first changed his diaper. My milk came in, I expressed it, and by the end of the first week they gave it to Aaron by a nasogastric tube. That was a momentous day! I was finally doing something for my baby that only *I* could do.

On the ninth day, it was time for me to leave the hospital. The thought of returning home without my baby was oppressive. When leaving time came, my husband practically had to pull me out of the hospital. I felt terribly empty in my maternity clothes, and in our apartment, where everything looked so different. My only thoughts were for Aaron. Within a few hours, I made the first of many walks back to the hospital. For the next two weeks I spent practically all day in the ICN. It became a second home to me. I no longer felt alien amidst the life-supporting machinery, or intimidated by the staff. I became part of the comradeship that existed there. Some of the mothers became familiar; we would share our experiences and our concerns. They alone really knew what I was going through.

During those two weeks I learned much about my baby and his needs; but most of all, I learned about myself. Although Aaron showed progress, he also had several setbacks. Each was a struggle for me to accept. The most frustrating were those directly affecting our mother-child relationship, such as problems with nursing. Many infants are able and eager to nurse immediately following birth, but my child wasn't able to nurse until he was ten days old. And even then, he certainly wasn't eager. Aaron was a preemie and therefore did not have the well-developed sucking reflex of full-term babies. He had to be taught. And the setting was less than

293

perfect: we would sit in a supply closet, where the heat was un-bearable and where the staff paraded in and out. I was depressed because I handled him awkwardly and couldn't relax. Even though the staff was supportive, emphasizing that it was an expected prob-lem with preemies, it was hard not to feel inadequate.

Another obstacle was the regression in Aaron's condition. Dur-ing the second week Aaron made such rapid improvement that we were told he might come home that weekend. But then he devel-oped recurrent periods where his heart and breathing rates would slow dramatically or stop, postponing the homecoming date. I felt like a Ping Pong ball — my hopes bouncing up and down as the end of the hospitalization would come into sight, only to fade away.

Eventually Aaron made it home healthy, and I could finally be his primary caretaker. But emotionally I had more work to do. Months later, while visiting old friends who recently had given birth, the discussion of their experiences forced me to recognize just how much I felt I had missed. Can you imagine longing to feel labor pains? I did. I also believed that I had missed out on one of the most important events of my life — watching my child being born. Once I admitted that loss, I was able to mourn it and to accept it. I stopped feeling like less of a mother. Aaron's birth was not something I could control. I can't change what happened. But I can accept it and be thankful that he is now healthy.

For some anxious months I was concerned about Aaron's de-velopment. I was supposed to adjust for "corrected" age, that is, to expect developmental tasks to occur in relation to his due date, rather than his birth date. But that was difficult to remember when my child was four months old and not yet demonstrating a social smile, or just beginning to show signs of head control. Fortunately, although Aaron started developing slowly, he has since progressed beautifully.

My road to motherhood has been difficult, and certainly totally different from how I had planned it would be. It began with my life threatened and the survival of my child questioned. But in spite of this, or maybe because of it, I am very close to Aaron and comfort-able mothering him.

Until her son's birth, DALE FRIEDLAND DANIELS was a social worker. She has elected to stay at home with Aaron for now. Dale and her family live in Philadelphia.

18

*Mothering Children
with Special Needs*

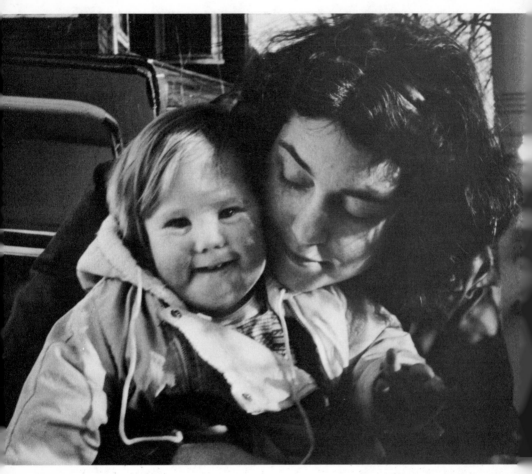

Robert Beck Stuhlmann

The Rainbow Child:
Living with a Down's Syndrome Child

TESS BECK STUHLMANN

We were overjoyed by the apparent healthiness of our premature infant. Over his face passed myriad expressions as he gazed intently into our eyes. We had worried about his breathing being fully developed, so it was wonderful to see his slow, easy, first breaths.

Christopher (Tuffy) was born in the caul. It's good luck, they say. A person born thus will never drown.

Into our bliss blundered the doctor, looking very nervous and rushed, a worried expression pursing his brow. "But there is something wrong with the baby," he blurted out, even before he had fully entered the room. I will never forget the way Bob's face fell instantly from ecstasy to despair. I didn't believe him. I said, "No, look, see — he's perfect."

The doctor quickly examined Christopher all over, turning back his ears, which were folded over like a puppy dog's. That was the only strange thing that I could see about him, and it didn't seem to merit such extreme concern.

The doctor then mumbled something which I only half heard about "this" being the cause of the early birth and the difficult and erratic labor. Then he said, "Maybe a little mongolism, I don't know." I hardly listened to him: I thought he was crazy. The baby looked adorable to me, and a fierce desire to protect him from this probing doctor seized me.

"Well, we love him just the same," I said to the nurse, "no matter what."

After the doctor delivered the placenta and stitched up a long tear, we were left alone with one another for a few hours while awaiting a particular pediatrician who was to examine our baby. It was a terribly conflicted time, with worry and joy intermingled; and I saw pain warring with pride in Bob's face as he gazed down at his first-born son in his arms. I was half in shock and half disbelieving that anything could be wrong with our baby.

The nurse took Tuffy to be checked by the pediatrician, and he confirmed that Christopher had Down's syndrome. He was very specific and careful in the way he explained it to us; I remember, even in my shock and pain, appreciating his consideration of our feelings. He also told us that Down's syndrome children are usually very easy babies, and that he had a cousin with such a child who was very happy. But it seemed too terrible to bear. I looked at the baby as the doctor held him up to show us how limply he hung down. I then heard the doctor say, "Many of these children have heart defects and do not survive long." And I looked at my son and hoped that he would die quickly.

I wanted to run away from this nightmare. I didn't want any part of him. Somehow Bob and I stumbled down the corridor to our room, collapsed into each other's arms, and wept inconsolably.

———————

The three days after Tuffy's birth were the worse — a thick, endless, heavy blanket of time through which I struggled merely to survive. I remember one helpful moment when a friend, an Episcopal priest, and his wife came and sat with us. They have a profoundly retarded boy of their own. Their presence and extraordinary quality of empathy was a rock to which we clung. I remember also that the nurses and hospital personnel were kind and allowed us space to be with our pain.

I was a kaleidoscope of incredibly intense feelings. I cried almost constantly. It was agony to be separated from Bob; I know what the Bible means when it says, "They shall become one flesh"; that is not a symbol but a reality. Bob and I felt bound together by a single skin of pain. It was painful to be near the baby, yet more painful to be away from him. He did not seem to need me at all. He just lay in his isolet and slept and slept, looking so pathetically frail and tiny. He weighed six pounds but was very skinny. I was sure that he was just going to fade away. A vast emptiness filled me. My heart yearned toward him — he was my baby, my longed-for treasure. My heart recoiled from him — he was an alien creature, surely none of my doing. I felt as if I had given birth to a baby, and that the baby had died. He had died. That vibrant, strong, healthy young man of our dreams who would be his daddy's pride and joy — follow in his footsteps to college — that tall young man who would some day tower over me and tease me by twirling me around, who would be intelligent and able to change a world so much in need of it . . . that child was dead. I had lost a child and yet had a real child's demands to meet. I was drained.

I felt that by having this "nonnormal" baby I had proved myself unworthy of anyone's respect, friendship, or interest. It was very important to hear from those who loved me, that they still loved me just the same. We could not think of an appropriate middle name for Christopher; we thought of grandparents' names, friends' names, but nothing seemed right. Although it was never said, I know that I felt that any one of them might be insulted by having their name given to a Down's child.

We agonized also over what it would be like in the future for Tuffy's sister to grow up with a retarded brother. Our images were of a very retarded person with strange mannerisms and no social skills.

The back of Christopher's head was almost flat. I hated it. I thought that there was no brain to push it out. And there was excess skin on his neck. I thought that it would be taken up if his brain were big enough. It disgusted me, and I felt ashamed of my feelings. I tried to hold him in positions where these symptoms did not show. I loved and hated him at the same time. I wanted to trade him for another baby, a "real" baby, the baby I had worked so hard to create.

When I was pregnant and friends speculated as to whether I was having a boy or girl, I used to say laughingly: "I can be sure of only one thing: it's a person!" Now I felt that I had somehow done the unthinkable — produced a nonhuman, a monster. And I had let Bob down: I had wanted to re-create the beauty of our love in a beautiful child. When I looked at Christopher, it was as if two photographs of two babies were superimposed one on the other, constantly shifting, so that first one appeared real, then the other. One was a strange, deformed, limp little creature, pathetic and repellent. The other was a frail, delicate rainbow child, miraculous in his completeness, rosy and peaceful. Of course, the child did not change; the shifting was all within me.

One of the initial effects of hearing the diagnosis was an inordinate concern for Tuffy's health. Although the diagnostic pediatrician had said to treat him like any healthy boy, he had also run down a list of problems many Down's children have or develop easily. We thought of Tuffy as very frail and wanted him carefully examined by the pediatrician assigned by the hospital. But she examined him perfunctorily, handling him as if he were an infected piece of meat that she did not want to contaminate herself by touching. I was furious, yet so insecure that I was unsure of my right to that fury. She asked,"You have been told already that something is not right with this baby?" We nodded, and she continued abruptly, "You do not have to keep a child like this. There are places . . ." I was outraged by her callousness. I drew myself together and with a great sense of dignity I told her that we would take our baby home and give him what love was in our hearts to give. I was disgusted by her attitude, and relieved when she left.

The only good thing about that episode was that the doctor's insensitive handling woke the baby so completely that he really cried for the first time; it was a relief to know he knew how. Then he nursed vigorously and long without any encouragement. In the beginning, every normal baby act of his was a gift to us.

I could not forget our doctor's obvious shock right after the birth, as if there were something terrible about our baby. The echo of his words lingered for a long time. I was very conscious that I had given birth to someone socially unacceptable. I thought Christopher was an embarrassment to everyone who came in contact with him, and I felt responsible for their embarrassment. I had to struggle with fear every time I took him to church, a store, or a friend's house. I also had to learn to be in need of help instead of always being the helping person. I called an Early Intervention program and requested a visitor. The most helpful advice she gave me was to allow myself to feel negative about Tuffy's Down's syndrome, that it didn't mean that I didn't love him.

———————

Tuffy brings a sense of joy with him wherever he goes. He has always had an extraordinary ability to connect with other people. I never realized before how closely I equated a person's intellect with his or her self-worth. I know now that our intellect, however wondrous a gift it may be, is *not* what makes us human. Tuffy may be retarded intellectually and developmentally, but emotionally and spiritually he is not retarded at all.

I had the mistaken idea that lack of character goes along with retardation. Not so: Christopher is aware, affectionate, independent, imaginative, creative, and a delight to be around. I wouldn't trade his "Down's-ness" for all the intelligence in the world.

When I feel negative about Tuffy's retardation, I am thinking of him abstractly and categorizing him as a type, a nonperson. Most of the time I feel good about him because I am responding to him as an individual, as himself.

———

We play a game in our family called "Essences" in which we say what kind of flower a person would be if she or he were a flower; or what kind of bird, etc. This is what I came up with for Christopher's essences when he was about nine months old:

He is like rainbow-colored soap bubbles
    or a piece of honey cake with whipped cream
Like a koala bear,
    or a pink rose wide open with its golden
        center held lovingly up to the sun,
Like a bee nuzzling to the nectar of my nipple,
    gorging himself in cozy abandonment,
He is full of paradoxes, yet totally open, simple and sweet,
As refreshing as a light summer wind at dusk,
As shiny as an evening star, and as round as a peach.

TESS BECK STUHLMANN has a daughter, Genevieve, and a son, Christopher. Tess is basically a stay-at-home mother, who is pleased that her husband is also involved with the children.

A Dark Window: Institutionalizing a Down's Syndrome Child

JANE S. DAHLBERG

It never occurred to me that my baby would be anything but normal. When he was born and I held him, when he was brought to me for his first breast-feeding, when my friends gathered in the hospital room and exclaimed over his resemblance to his father, I glowed with joy. We had his name chosen — my husband's name.

And then the pediatrician, an old friend, called and said that the baby wasn't doing well, and that I couldn't breast-feed him because he needed a special formula. While I was protesting, the obstetrician came in and quickly gave me a shot to dry up my milk. A moment later my husband came in with my suitcase, ready to take me home without the baby. As he hurried me out of the hospital, he explained, "I *need* you with me. Our two other children miss you. We'll come back to get the baby in a few days when he's stronger. No point in staying in the hospital; you can rest at home. Come right now. No need to get dressed. The car is downstairs."

There was no time either to think or to question. In a few moments I had switched from the role of exultant mother to that of a confused, hurried, mindless being. I allowed myself to be driven home and then whisked into bed. I loved and trusted my husband so much that I did not even think of questioning him.

Once I was safely in bed, he held me in his arms and told me that the baby was a mongoloid. He and the doctors had decided that we were not going to bring him home. They had planned my sudden departure from the hospital to spare me the agony of finding out while on the maternity ward. They had found a good home for the retarded where the baby would go.

I had no part in the decision save to accept it. Looking back, I'm glad now that I didn't have to choose; I could not have made that decision. Emotionally, physiologically, and psychologically, I was prepared for a baby. For days I didn't do very much except cry. I would awaken clutching at pillows as though they were babies. I could not go outside or even look out of the windows lest I see another baby. The hope of motherhood saw no light through the windows. Hope's windows were dark.

I longed for my baby. I wanted to hold him and to love him. So did my husband. He had made the painful decision that bringing him home would be wrong for us: we are both professional people and we would have had to change our lives completely to bring up a retarded child; our other children would have had their lives changed by having a retarded brother at home; a retarded child would have suffered ridicule and social isolation; and if we had brought him home and then decided later to institutionalize him, it would have been even more difficult. A strong-willed husband, a confused and ambivalent mother — the decision stood. Heart-broken, we suffered together in our pain. Nineteen years later we still cry sometimes.

In a situation like this one, no solution is "right" or "wrong." Decisions must be personal; there are no rules — only guaranteed heartache. Our consciences were eased somewhat by the discovery of a small, private home for the retarded not too far from our house. Although I had gone along with the decision, I was most afraid that my baby would not be loved. What we found was a staff of women devoting their lives to their charges, and loving them.

Many parents have kept their retarded children; and many have placed them in homes or institutions. I would not presume to tell anyone how to decide. I do know that my husband was right about how much more difficult it would have been to have given him up later.

For *all* parents a retardate is a tragedy, but the most tragic I have seen was a mother who brought her six-year-old son to the home. She sat near me watching him being led away and crying, "Mommy, Mommy." After six years of mothering she had to give him up because her husband could not bear their way of life: her choice was her son or her husband. After her son left the room, she fell on the floor sobbing and could not get up. I have seen her often since then, when we are both visiting at the home. Her separation from her son was far worse than mine. It was unbearably cruel, and she has continued to suffer bitterly.

———————

My husband and I have made a life for ourselves that barely includes our retarded son. Our work, our other two children, our home leave time for only occasional visits to him. Is that cruel? Heartless? At times I feel so guilty that I rush over to see him, which always delights him. He does, however, seem happy in the home where he has lived for nineteen years. He knows no other home, although we once tried bringing him to our house when he was younger. Unfortunately he cried when we returned him to the home and became difficult to handle. So we had to decide either to bring him to our house every weekend, or not to bring him at all. Again, it was a hard, unnatural decision. And again pragmatism won — professional life, other children, other obligations. I think he no longer remembers coming to our house, the house that is not his. A house with a dark window.

In his home he is with peers who are like him. He does not know that he is different or "special." No one laughs at him, stares at him, ostracizes him, is repulsed by him, or pities him. His life is ordered. He goes to school each day in the home, and there is no such thing as failure. He gets love, although not as much as I think I might have given him; he is loving, as are most people who have Down's syndrome; he has no worldly cares.

What have I learned that I can share with other mothers? That a normal child is precious. That life brings unexpected trials. That tragic choices are personal and cannot be judged by others. That living is filled with "might-have-beens," and there is no going back. And that what seems tragic is not always so.

Soon after our son was born, a friend remarked, "You have what every parent wants for a baby, a child who will always be happy." I believe that our son is happy — in a childish, Peter Pan kind of way. But like Peter Pan, he is without a mother. I try to be grateful for that happiness, although I all too often ache for the person he might have been. Hope has brought many lights into our house over the years, but there is always one window without a light — a dark window.

JANE S. DAHLBERG is a college dean living in New York City. She is married to her second husband and has three grown sons.

Coping with the Unexpected: Cerebral Palsy

LINDA ZACK

Starting at the beginning of a story is always best. Michael and I planned our child's birth very carefully. Six months prior to actually trying to conceive, I purposely went on a health kick to get my body and mind in the best possible condition and to assure our baby every opportunity of a healthy life. I even started jogging — up to forty miles a week at one point — until I finally reached my goal.

We conceived without problems. I continued to care for myself and our baby almost to the point of obsession, so that nothing would go wrong. My doctor allowed me to continue to jog, and I did so until my sixth month.

Noah was born precisely on my due date. My husband and I struggled through a twenty-three-hour labor and delivery. The baby was not moving down the birth canal fast enough, and eventually had to be delivered by forceps. We were overwhelmed with joy at the long-awaited entrance into our lives of a seven-and-a-half-pound baby boy. We were even happier when he scored a nine on the Apgar test, which records alertness and ease in breathing.

Noah seemed perfectly normal during his first few weeks of life. We were awake most of that time and so were aware of his every move: sleeping through the night was not one of his attributes.

Upon seeing six-week-old Noah at his first checkup, our pediatrician detected an extreme tightness in his hips and suggested that we consult with an orthopedist. I was somewhat concerned but also pleased to see that my doctor examined him very thoroughly in order to rule out any serious conditions.

Although the orthopedist felt that Noah's problems were confined to a tightness in his leg and hip regions only, no one is more in touch with a child's mental and physical progress than a mother, and somehow I knew that my child's problems were more complicated than "tight hips and legs." By that time, I was beginning to feel that Noah's development was *more* than normally slow. He was, I believed, very delayed.

When Noah was eight months old, I was still frustrated because of little visible improvement and decided to get another opinion. This time the doctor gave me three possible reasons for the tightness: dislocated hip; displacement of the hip; and cerebral palsy. The doctor believed that it was not cerebral palsy and that Noah, in fact, had a displaced hip. He stated that if this were his child, he would have had him in braces four months ago.

Both orthopedists believed the problem was not neurological. The tragic fact is that both orthopedists were wrong.

When Noah was a year old, my pediatrician suggested that we do further testing — this time neurological. It seemed that Noah's head size had not grown in proportion with his body since he was six months old. The fear of my earlier suspicions crept slowly but surely into our lives. I was frightened but felt that it would be a relief to know if indeed there was a neurological reason for Noah's problems. A week later, after extensive testing, we got the word that Noah in fact had cerebral palsy. The doctor said that his legs and arms were affected. He would walk, but the doctor could not say when. He also said that Noah would probably be a slow learner and that mental retardation was a possibility. He then walked us to the door, after making some recommendations, and casually said, "Good-bye."

We were devastated. What, we wondered, had we done wrong? Had the doctors made a terrible mistake? It just could not be possible! What had happened to our perfect little baby? What would the future bring for him? Why him? Why us?

────────────

The first day was spent as if we were in mourning. We knew very little about cerebral palsy. We pictured the most severe cases we had seen on television, or on posters. The day seemed endless. We hoped that we would wake up and discover that it had been a bad dream. We anxiously awaited a phone call from one of our doctors to help us deal with the nightmare. No one phoned. For days, no one phoned. I was so upset, so helpless, so alone.

I was feeling dejected, and rather than wallow in self-pity, I needed to take action. I needed desperately to reach out for help, so

I took the initiative and spent the first two weeks after the diagnosis calling people. I started with my community facilities, which had wonderful people, close by, ready and willing to help us get through our ordeal.

Then I spent many days and nights researching people who work with cerebral palsied children, finding the best treatment for Noah, as well as evaluations of the facilities accessible to us. It was a lot of work, and I know I'll be spending many more days and nights trying to find the answers; but he is my child, and he deserves to have every possible chance for a normal, productive, fulfilling life. It really is up to the parents to turn every stone, and I will.

The hardest part is accepting the fact that somewhere, sometime, something went terribly wrong. What is miraculous is that I have somehow developed a tremendous inner strength, probably because my child's mental and physical health depend upon it. In spite of depression or frustration, I must persevere.

It is now three months since Noah was diagnosed as having cerebral palsy. We are not convinced, given the varying doctors' opinions and tests, that anyone truly knows the extent of or even the precise afflictions that our son has incurred. He is a happy, sociable baby who feels no abnormal physical pain. Through the specialized therapy sessions set up for him at home twice weekly, he is making slow but positive progress with his motor delays. Every inkling of development is received by me as a milestone. I get great pleasure from seeing his slight progress; he brings me a tremendous amount of joy.

It may be years before we know the actual extent of the brain damage; both we and the doctors believe that sometime around the actual birth, brain damage did occur. Ours, then, is a waiting game. It is not easy, but we work very hard at keeping our lives as "normal" as possible. When all is said and done, we tend to become philosophical as to why these things happen. I do and must believe that there is a reason, even if only to make me take inventory of my life, and I believe that through this ordeal the quality of our lives has changed for the better. What used to be important to me before the crisis has changed profoundly: I spend a great deal of my time on the telephone, always searching for new programs and facilities, or for someone to enlighten me on how to deal with the situation.

While doctors can and should play an important role in helping parents connect with all the useful organizations, my doctors failed to extend themselves by contacting these organizations on my behalf, leaving me helpless. In my most urgent time of need, the doctors simply were not there for me. I still have a bitter taste in my mouth for the detached, unsympathetic manner in which the "professionals" conducted themselves. I wish that they saw their jobs as going beyond clinical diagnosis. A simple phone call would have made such a difference during those indescribably painful first days.

We are taking one day at a time. If we look too far into the future, it seems overwhelmingly bleak. I can only suggest that if you are the mother of a special-needs child, you should enjoy your child just as he or she is, and give him or her the best that you can, in spite of the handicap.

We have learned that we must also continue to fulfill our needs as husband and wife, and as individuals. It's so easy to lose oneself and so crucial for all involved to retain a clear sense of self. I am not afraid to feel depressed, cheated, or guilty. These are normal responses from which I was able to derive strength. Yet he is my baby, and I love him. He's playful and happy, and for us he's perfect.

LINDA ZACK and her English-born husband, Michael, have been married for five-and-one-half "good years," and live in Brookline, Massachusetts. She is a part-time dental hygienist and travel agent.

Mothering a Gifted Child

CAROLYN CAMPBELL

A gifted child. The description calls to mind Einstein, Edison, and twelve-year-olds in college. I have come to see giftedness, however, as a very mixed blessing.

Before Aaron was two, he knew the alphabet. He could also count past twenty. At two and a half, he began reading. I did not teach him to read. In fact, I only recall reading to him once or twice. By the time I thought he would be interested, he was already doing it on his own. Now, at three and a half, he sounds out and reads words such as *metamorphosis, automatic, vinegar,* and *San Francisco.*

When the number 100,000 flashed across our television screen recently, he read it correctly. It is hard for me to think of a word that he cannot read. I doubt that he always understands the meaning, but he pronounces every word perfectly.

At first, I didn't think Aaron was unusual. I assumed that because I was a librarian and constantly brought books home, he was following in my footsteps and simply enjoyed reading. At the grocery store, as we strolled through the produce section, he looked at the signs and clearly said "vegetables," "fruit," or "potatoes."

Soon after he began reading, people would comment to me about it excitedly. I still felt uncertain as to his giftedness, yet professors, teachers, counselors, and mothers of other children who have tested as "gifted" have assured me that he is. The usual formula statement is, "If he could read at two, then he is gifted." I haven't had him tested because I have been told that it is difficult to find someone to test a three-year-old anyway, and that testing before the age of four is both inconclusive and a traumatic experience for children and parents. I feel most comfortable with one professor's evaluation: "Let's say he's doing things most three-year-olds don't do," she said. "Even the label 'gifted' is not always a help." However, I do sometimes wish that I had a definite measure that could provide conclusive proof. On the other hand, I was more comfortable before I realized that Aaron was special. There is security knowing that your child is progressing at the same rate as all the others.

I often feel alone as the mother of a gifted child. His intellectual development is markedly different from that of his friends, and there are no charts I can measure him by. Most child-care books contain only a scant, vague section on giftedness.

And I get very little support from other mothers. In fact, their reactions are often disturbing. "What have you done for him?" they ask, staring me coldly in the face. "What courses have you enrolled him in? What tests has he been given? Did you sit and read with him every night to get him that way?"

My greatest uncertainty *is* what I should do for my son. He does have special needs. How will a child who has sounded out *metamorphosis* feel about reading *See Jane run*? I have visions of his losing interest in school. I worry about his attempting to remain at the level of his friends when he could be far beyond them.

Our school district does not have funds for a special gifted program, or for students who want to start kindergarten before the age of five. Socially my son is still very much a three-year-old, crying for Mommy when he falls, putting his pants on backwards, and having a temper tantrum on occasion. I cannot picture him in kindergarten, even if he is mentally ready.

I have considered attending a private preschool with Aaron because I feel very inept about stimulating and encouraging him properly. But I believe that pushing him to read faster would be wrong. Reading is something he's already mastered, and I should work with him on other areas.

In general, I am trying to tone down the academic side of him, trying to help him enjoy being the child that he still is. I am placing emphasis on typical children's activities, and I try to give him the same recognition for participation in these that I do when he reads. I am also following the advice of a teacher and attempting to broaden his language arts experience, the area where his particular giftedness seems to lie. We have "plays" at home in which we are each a character acting out actions and consequences. We play word games, and I am teaching him Spanish. He also likes a modified form of Scrabble.

I have found that I can't discuss his giftedness with most mothers. Some feel threatened by Aaron. They think that I am bragging, or merely exaggerating. I can tell that they think that by "reading" I must mean looking at the pictures and talking about them. Or they call it coincidence. "Did he just happen to see a few letters and put them together?" Their defenses make me both sad and angry. I find myself having to prove my son's talents by finding the longest word in existence and having him read it to them.

It even reaches the point where I feel like placing their child next to mine and asking them both to read words from a magazine. I often ask friends, "Did you see how much clearer Aaron talked, or higher Aaron counted, or faster Aaron read than so-and-so's child?" And then I dislike myself for this display of my own lack of security and need for reinforcement. Also, I ask myself why I should be offended that certain mothers insist that my child is normal and average.

I never wish that Aaron were not gifted. I see nurturing as a difficult task where the reward is proportional to the effort invested. Yes, he is more difficult to stimulate and to challenge. But there is much more ability there to challenge; he can go much further.

If I can help him overcome his differentness and keep him excited about learning, I believe he will have far greater opportunity and scope than my husband and I ever did. His potential excites me. I feel I was given a great challenge when I was blessed with my son. I fantasize about the colleges he might attend, and the careers he might seek.

I think of Aaron's unusual capabilities in relation to my second son too. I worry about people comparing the two of them. Already people ask if Chris has shown signs of reading or giftedness. Chris seems less intellectual and less dynamic than Aaron. Where Aaron is forceful, Chris is calm. Perhaps Aaron will feel driven to set the world on fire, and Chris will be content to watch him do it. I have the feeling that their abilities will even out eventually.

Aaron is a child whose brain has somehow moved ahead of the rest of his development; he's out of balance. He's ready to learn and think, yet he still has a hard time putting his arm through a long-sleeved turtleneck. I hate to see him frustrated by the different levels of his own personality, a problem other children experience less than he does.

My greatest wish is to encourage him properly in his potential, to help *both* of us see his giftedness as a two-sided entity which requires foresight and patience. I must see not only that he is stimulated and excited about developing further, but also that he remains a happy child.

CAROLYN CAMPBELL and her family live in South Sandy, Utah. She is a librarian and freelance writer.

19

When
Things Go Wrong

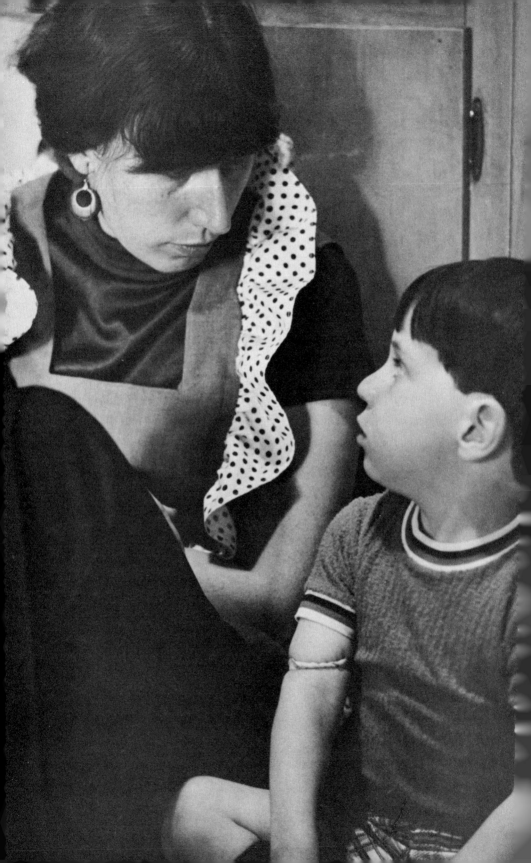

Major Surgery on Our Six-Week-Old Child

RONNIE FRIEDLAND

The wave of contentment, joy, and delight on which I coasted after my son's birth crashed abruptly one month later when I learned that he had a medical problem requiring major surgery. Suddenly the world was divided into healthy versus unhealthy families and lucky versus unlucky people, and we were on the wrong side.

At the usual one-month checkup, our pediatrician uncomfortably informed me that he believed our son had a serious problem. He advised having Joshua x-rayed immediately to confirm his diagnosis of a birth defect. I reacted with shock, disbelief, and anger. Initially I was even unwilling to expose my son to x-rays, based on what I thought was a bizarre diagnosis, but I was finally convinced of the need.

From our protected enclosure, my husband and I watched helplessly as the x-ray machine loomed over our son's tiny body. We couldn't help chuckling with pride when our four-week-old infant managed to push and kick aside the lead pillows intended to restrain his arms and legs. The entire episode was, however, a painful initiation into the limitations of parenthood and the separateness of our child. We learned that Joshua's body would have its own experiences and that we could not protect him from them. His life was his own.

The x-rays confirmed the pediatrician's diagnosis, and we were then sent to a "pediatric neurosurgeon," a title I found ominous. The waiting room shocked and depressed me; it was filled with child after child with shaved heads and scars, some brain damaged, some not. I was horrified that *our* child belonged there. I felt I had entered a kind of nether world populated with children normally not seen. I could foresee our lives changing, our interests becoming medical. Already far off in the unrecoverable distance was the world of healthy, normal children. I was in a situation I had previously feared even to contemplate.

The neurosurgeon told us that in my second month of pregnancy, for some unknown, nongenetic reason, the connecting tissue around one of the bones in the soft spot of Joshua's head had closed prematurely, preventing his skull from growing properly. Unlike the other bones in his soft spot, the closing of this one did not endanger the brain. The problem was purely "cosmetic": without surgery our son would look extremely strange; his forehead would have an increasingly large ridge. And even with surgery there was no guarantee how "normal" he would ever appear.

As the neurosurgeon talked to us, my mind drifted back to all those nights when I had sat nursing Joshua, looking lovingly at him, and gradually noticed a small ridge in his forehead. I would look at his otherwise perfect face and fantasize that the ridge would somehow disappear. I tried to convince myself that it was something all infants had and that I simply had never looked closely enough. Each morning I somehow "forgot" to mention this observation to my husband. And although I had intended to ask the pediatrician about it, I again "forgot." Even when he recognized a problem, I failed to connect it with those late-night observations — such was the strength of my wish to deny them.

Once the diagnosis was confirmed, my brain felt numbed and my body ill. I had been on an extraordinary high, utterly enamored of my son and of my husband. The drop to my present distress was enormous. The most difficult part was accepting that this sweet, innocent infant, whose slightest cough was of such concern to me, had a serious problem. It seemed terribly unfair. While at first I felt chiefly shock and disbelief, gradually bitterness and despair emerged. Why Joshua? I wondered. Why me?

Beyond that, I was saddened that Joshua would be deprived of the joyous environment we had so gladly provided. It was late in June, and Dan was on vacation from teaching until September. We had expected to spend the whole summer together, giving Joshua the unusual opportunity to have both parents constantly available. We would still both be there, but the atmosphere would be charged with tension, tinged with sadness.

My husband was endlessly supportive, loving, and understanding through this ordeal. His encouragement and mere presence were crucial for me at that time. He was able to cope with his own anxieties and to provide support for me as well. We were fortunate that the crisis solidified our relationship, uniting us in our love both for our child and for each other.

The two-week wait between the diagnosis and the surgery seemed endless. I was exhausted from caring for our infant and still weak from a difficult delivery. Having enough energy to cope with the extra strain became a prime concern. I worried that Joshua would suffer psychological damage from undergoing surgery so early, that he would think of life as painful and traumatic. However, we were reassured by psychologists that he was too young to understand or remember much, and that as long as I could remain with him in the hospital there would be no harmful psychological consequences.

My main fear was that I would lose my son, that he would not survive the surgery. Any major surgery performed on a six-week-old child is dangerous because of the anesthesia. And so, although the actual surgical procedure was relatively straightforward, there were serious risks. As these might be my last days with my son, I felt that I should make the most of them; but it was difficult. Warring within me were two contradictory impulses: one to withdraw from Joshua to protect myself in case I lost him; the other to love him as much as I could while I still had him.

The day we had to hospitalize Joshua was a nightmare. I cried as I registered him, knowing what lay in store. Entering pediatrics and seeing all the very sick children further depressed me. Once we were given a room, countless blood tests and repetitive examinations by practicing residents followed. How I hated to have them looking for what was wrong with this child I adored. I tried hard to treat Joshua as lovingly and as normally as possible, so that he would not be upset by all the changes. And I felt relieved that the crisis was finally coming to a resolution.

Although the neurosurgeons we consulted had convinced me that the operation was necessary, as the time approached I grew increasingly unsure. Was a normal appearance worth the risk of loss of life? Each doctor we spoke to had treated us coldly, impersonally, and with condescension. Despite repeated questions, it had been difficult to elicit any information from any of them — beginning with the pediatrician who made himself unavailable to us after the diagnosis and including several neurosurgeons. Finally, the night before the surgery, a neurologist who came to examine Joshua was able to address our feelings and to satisfy our need to know more. He reassured me that it would be too cruel to Joshua not to have the operation, too cruel to deny him a normal life. Talking with him gave me the courage to sign the release allowing the operation to occur — an awesome responsibility.

That night I stayed in Joshua's room, silently staring at his peacefully sleeping face, trying to memorize the features I might never see alive again.

—————

We had been told not to go to the hospital during the surgery, but to wait in our room for a call from the neurosurgeon immediately afterward. Hours after it was supposed to be over we were still waiting. Finally the surgeon called to say, casually, that all was fine.

Once our greatest fear — loss of life — was past, new problems arose. I ached to hold Joshua in his favorite position, with his forehead against my chest and his little body all curled up against me, bottom sticking out in the air. But holding him at all had become exceedingly dangerous. As most of the bone in his forehead had been removed, I had to be sure not to touch or bump his head. For three months, until the bone grew back in his forehead, we could not even wash it! Although joyful that I could hold him again, I froze as my arms approached his bandaged head, petrified that I would inadvertently do him permanent damage. Yet I had to master my fears and my desire to avoid a difficult situation; my child needed me.

Joshua spent the next three days in intensive care. Had I not been nursing him, I would have been permitted to be with him only infrequently during the day and not at all during the night. Because he was breast-feeding, however, the nurses would call me in our rented room across the street (I slept whenever he did) as soon as he began to stir, and I would be by his side moments after he awakened. Although I hadn't especially enjoyed nursing until then (it wasn't the overwhelmingly wonderful experience I had hoped for), I was delighted to have something I could do to make him feel better, and therefore very grateful I had nursed.

Joshua recovered very quickly from the surgery, and we were

able to leave the hospital on the third day. Although his shaved, scarred, and stitched head was as shocking to others as the children in the waiting room had been to us, we proudly took pictures, finding him beautiful. But one of the most painful issues after the surgery was coping with other people's reactions to our son's appearance. I'll always remember a distant acquaintance who peeked into the baby carriage when Joshua still had plastic stitches lining his head, then looked up at us in dismay and bewilderment and, not knowing what to say, mumbled something and raced off. How I feel for mothers who have to bear those agonies always.

We were frequently faced with new emergencies during the next three months — Joshua went through a dangerous phase of hitting his forehead with his fists and we had to be constantly on the alert to intercept — but we were able to handle them fairly well once the central issue of survival was no longer in question.

Especially at the beginning of the crisis, the outpouring of support we received from our friends and family was extremely helpful. It partially bridged — even though only a bit — that painful gap separating us (unlucky people) from them, making us feel less tainted and alone. Nevertheless, while I had previously turned to friends when in trouble, I felt this "blood" matter required family. My parents provided invaluable support during the ordeal. They instinctively knew to treat Joshua exactly as they would have if nothing were wrong — a wonderful tonic.

I was surprised to observe that however painful the knowledge was that I had produced an "imperfect" child, I spent little time and energy dwelling on it. What most concerned me was Joshua and what he would suffer, not what it meant about me as a mother. And however hard I tried to feel responsible and blame myself, going over everything I ate or drank during my pregnancy, it somehow did not feel real. Finally I accepted that no one was to blame: it had just happened. And yet, on another level, I came up with the explanation that I had been guilty of hubris, feeling too joyful and confident. I had exceeded my quota of happiness, and something had to happen to take it away, to even things out. Although irrational, the explanation is still convincing.

Whereas at the time of the diagnosis we felt singled out and resentful, we now feel relatively lucky. We were fortunate that the problem was not chronic, that it was remedied through surgery.

Our ordeal was finite; the results were cosmetically good. No one would ever guess what Joshua went through as an infant, and he has retained his exuberant disposition.

Although we are back on the side of the lucky families, a sense of our vulnerability and of the fragility of good health has never left me. The experience has made me tougher, better able to cope with any new crisis that may lie ahead. And I know that all the love in the world can't safeguard Joshua from experiencing his allotment of pain in life.

Conquering Infertility

MIRIAM MORGAN

Until last March, when I found out that I was at last pregnant after almost three-and-a-half years of trying to conceive, I had felt I was the victim of some great cosmic joke. My husband Rick and I had never had much interest in children during the first few years of our marriage — we were both too busy with our careers, mine in teaching and his in medicine, and we enjoyed our free time together.

Then, after about five years of marriage, when I was twenty-seven and Rick twenty-nine, I began to think that the time might be right. With Rick's half-hearted agreement, I went off the Pill.

After a few months had elapsed and I hadn't become pregnant or gotten my period, I went to my doctor for a checkup. (To make matters worse, my regular gynecologist had moved and I was in the process of trying to find another doctor with whom I could feel as comfortable. I had gone through about five of them before I had found a good one in the first place.)

Initially my new doctor didn't foresee any fertility problem, but put me on a medication called Provera to help bring on my period. He also instructed me to begin taking my basal body temperature daily to determine my "most fertile" time of the month. I thought there should be more he could do, but I was told repeatedly the workup for infertility does not begin until a couple has been trying to conceive for one year, especially when the woman has been on the Pill for several years, as I had been. The doctors assume that it takes a year for your body to overcome the effects of that nasty medication.

I continued to take my temperature every morning during the next few weeks and months — a horrible daily reminder that something was wrong. During my three years of trying to conceive, I must have broken at least a half-dozen of those thermometers in frustration and resentment.

As time passed, my frustration changed into fear and self-doubt. I was afraid that something was wrong with me physically or mentally. Since the doctors say that the psyche plays a major role in fertility problems, I started to wonder: Am I neurotic? A child hater? Do I despise my own body? Do I despise my mother? What was it? Did this mean I wasn't ready to become a mother?

I shared some of these feelings with one or two close friends, but not with any members of my family. I didn't want to upset them, and even more important, I wanted to spare myself their questions. I did not feel at all comfortable discussing such a personal problem at this point. My parents and in-laws would often ask when, or if, we intended to have children, and give us well-intentioned advice about not being "old parents." Later, when I did tell them about our fertility problems, they provided much-needed support.

After a few more months, my periods began to come on their own, so I discontinued taking the Provera. Aha, I thought. It just took my body a while to regulate itself after taking the birth-control pill for so many years. Now everything is functioning normally and surely I'll conceive shortly. But, as each period arrived on schedule, I felt my confidence evaporate and my level of tension and anxiety rise. I again blamed myself for having an "improper" mental attitude toward conception, for I was sure all the difficulties were "in my head." Of course, this in turn heightened my anxiety. A vicious spiral was beginning.

Finally my doctor began the diagnostic workup for infertility. The first step was to analyze Rick's semen. The result: the semen analysis indicated low to borderline fertility. Strike one.

Although both of us were upset with the test result, I also felt relieved. At least there was a real physical, as opposed to psychological, reason for our infertility. And there were surgical methods to correct the problem.

The surgery is relatively minor, but there is no guarantee that it will be successful. And even if it is, it takes about six months before the sperm count can stabilize and a new count is reliable.

While Rick's repeat semen analysis six months after the operation still was abnormal, both his urologist and my gynecologist felt that it had improved enough to indicate that conception was possible.

During the few months following the surgery, my mood improved dramatically. There had been a relatively straightforward physical problem, and it had been diagnosed and corrected. Now surely everything would be okay.

But it was not. When I still was not pregnant ten months later, the possibility of another problem arose. My basal body temperature chart did not show the classic ovulatory pattern, so I had to undergo a very painful procedure called an endometrial biopsy, to determine whether or not ovulation had taken place. I was not prepared for the piercing pain of the procedure, but at least it was brief, and I was assured it would not have to be repeated. In what seems to have been the pattern of our situation, the lab report on the biopsy was ambiguous; therefore we had to assume that I was not ovulating. Strike two.

At this point, the whole mess began to seem like a bad joke. No one else I knew had ever had such problems trying to get pregnant; rather, everyone was trying to avoid becoming pregnant! Why wasn't I ovulating? What was wrong with my body? Was my mental state causing these physical problems?

I never was able to answer those questions, but I began to accept the fact that, again, at least there was a physical abnormality that was potentially correctable.

After discussion with my doctor, we decided I should begin

medication to induce ovulation. I took a mild fertility drug, Clomid, for five days each month while continuing to take my temperature each morning. In addition, Rick and I were told that we should have intercourse every other night. That kind of schedule put a great strain on spontaneous lovemaking. Often we both felt, Oh no, not again!

Each month when I got my period, it was a bitter letdown. I had to have monthly pelvic exams to make sure that the Clomid had not produced cysts (one of its possible side effects). Sitting in the doctor's waiting room surrounded by fertile women with big bellies made me more and more depressed. In fact, I got depressed seeing a pregnant woman anywhere; I tried to keep this feeling in the background, consciously thinking about my situation as little as possible. My friends continued to be extremely supportive.

The dosage of Clomid was increased twice within the next few months; still I did not become pregnant. The doctor decided it was necessary to repeat one of those painful biopsies even though I had been assured I would not have to go through it again. I was very nervous, but this time I took tranquilizers and had Rick come with me. That helped — it wasn't as bad as the first time.

The lab report was somewhat more positive, indicating that I probably was ovulating with the Clomid. The next step was to determine whether the Fallopian tubes were open or blocked. This was to be done with a hysterosalpingogram, in which dye is injected and then followed through the Fallopian tubes with x-rays, indicating whether the tubes are open.

Meanwhile Rick accepted a new job offer, and we were getting ready to move back to California. We planned a two-month round-the-country vacation coincident with the move, and decided it would be better to wait until we were settled into our new home before proceeding with the hysterosalpingogram. Besides, maybe I would become pregnant during our vacation: the infertility could stem from psychological causes, and maybe the change of pace was what we needed.

After a fabulous trip, but no pregnancy, we moved into our new home. That occupied most of my time and energy. During our travels I had been off the Clomid; we had decided with my doctor that since I couldn't be checked for cysts each month it would be better to stop any medication for a while.

323

When I felt somewhat settled and organized, I reestablished contact with my initial doctor who, coincidentally, was now in practice not far from our new home. We decided to proceed at once with the hysterosalpingogram. It showed a blockage of both Fallopian tubes. Strike three.

When my doctor told me the results of the test, I just couldn't believe it: What had I ever done to deserve this? Why us? Why me? And what had caused the blockage?

Of course these questions had no answers — then or now. Rick and I tried logically, with the help of my doctor, to consider the alternatives. There were only two: either accept the fact that we probably would never have children; or undergo surgery to try to open the tubes.

The thought of surgery terrified me. The procedure was relatively simple, but the surgery was considered "major" — six to eight weeks for recovery. The success rate is fifty percent. I thought that sounded terrible, but evidently in medical circles it is considered very respectable. Even if the surgery is effective in reopening the tubes, they have a tendency to close back up after six months. There is also an increased chance of tubal pregnancy after the surgery, which would necessitate a hysterectomy. In short, there were no guarantees of anything positive.

Rick and I agonized over the decision for days. I was thoroughly depressed and panicked. On top of fear at the thought of a knife cutting into me, I was in a new community, with no close friends or relatives nearby for emotional support, and my husband was in a new job and himself somewhat insecure. In addition, I had interviewed for a very good job and felt sure that I would get it. But it was to start immediately, so I didn't want to be out of commission for eight weeks.

Despite everything, we opted for the surgery. After coming this far, I really didn't want to stop short of doing all that reasonably could be done. This would be the last step.

I did get the job I wanted, and the employer decided to hold it for me until after I had recovered. That gave me incentive to get back on my feet as soon as possible.

Right after the surgery I felt extremely high for a day or so, especially when my doctor said how well the procedure had gone and raised his estimate for success to seventy percent. But then I began to feel incredibly lousy, both mentally and physically. I found out later that this is a typical reaction to surgery, but it didn't help me to feel better at the time.

I did recover my strength within what was considered "normal" time, and began my new job about five weeks after surgery. Within another ten days or so, I got my period and began taking Clomid again to ensure ovulation. And once more I took my temperature each morning — breaking more thermometers in the process.

I grew anxious as each period arrived; I was very aware of the "six-month deadline," even though I knew that nothing in medicine was as exact or as certain as a "deadline." My doctor and my husband both remained optimistic and full of encouragement. And they were right. When my period was one week late, I began to hope. When it was two weeks late, I had the pregnancy test. Was I ever nervous that day waiting for the result. It was positive! I had it repeated to be certain. Then I had a sonogram to make sure the pregnancy wasn't tubal. It wasn't.

Now, at seven-and-one-half months, I am huge. Every time the baby kicks, I think it is a miracle.

MIRIAM MORGAN plans to deliver her child in an alternative birthing room in a San Francisco hospital. Miriam has been working part-time as a staff reporter for a daily suburban newspaper in California, and makes her home in San Mateo.

Coping with Infant Cancer

BRENDA G. STONE

Holding her snug against my breast in a circle of warmth and love, I ache. So newly departed from the shelter of my womb, so connected nutritionally through nursing, we have barely begun the normal process of separation. Yet I am forced to prepare for the reality that we may separate long before I am ready. Death has become real to me. Paradoxically, so has life.

Natalie's birth was magnificent — no drugs, husband coached, family present, plus all the elements for early mother-infant bonding. Although we have another child by adoption, Natalie was our first experience with pregnancy and birth. John and I were full of confidence that we had given this child the ideal start to a normal, healthy existence. Having battled infertility for years, we thought we had conquered the most difficult task of our lives.

Three-and-one-half months later, with no warning, we found ourselves in the throes of a life-and-death crisis. What we had believed to be a small cyst on Natalie's clitoris was in fact a malignant mass. After extensive tests of all her bones, liver, spleen, and bone marrow, we were told finally that she had neuroblastoma, cancer of the nervous tissues.

Prior to this I had no idea how difficult it was to grasp the tremendous amount of information thrown out rather quickly and nonchalantly by surgeons, pathologists, radiologists, and anesthesiologists ad infinitum. We struggled to educate ourselves, pored over medical texts, asked numerous questions, and became lay experts on neuroblastoma. Wanting to make wise decisions about Natalie's care, yet constantly finding ourselves in a game where we didn't know the rules, was frustrating and demoralizing. Ultimately we had no reasonable choice but to accept the judgment of medical professionals.

Surgery was the first step. Our tiny infant lay helpless in an operating room at the mercy of a surgeon whom we had known for only a few days. We knew that she would lose an adrenal gland along with the primary tumor, but discovering (after a four-hour ordeal) that her kidney had also been removed was a traumatic blow. In one short week we had been thrust from the blissful illusion of normalcy to the reality of mutilation and hovering death. John and I wept.

Amazingly, within a week after surgery, Natalie seemed happy and normal (a word which now has relative meaning for me). Her strength renewed ours.

Then began the second phase of her treatment. Frequent trips to various doctors, another hospitalization, radiotherapy, and daily observation of her progress imposed a different way of life upon all of us. I soon realized that maintaining any sort of regular, predictable routine would be impossible. The demand of managing her medical care forced me to delay completion of my work as a doctoral student. Initially, accepting that disappointment was not easy, but my values and priorities have gradually altered. The assumption that life flows and children flow with it has changed to a belief that life flows right through your fingers if you don't hang on to it. Now I attempt to hang on to each day, to embrace its purpose before it's gone. Fatigue, however, often overrides my intentions. Natalie has not slept well since surgery, and this has created an additional strain. Nevertheless, although I am tired and drained as I nurse her in the darkness, I cherish the opportunity to hold her and to express my love.

My emotions are constantly in flux. I feel as if I'm on a perpetual roller-coaster ride: just when I've reached the top I find myself catapulted into the next slump, only to emerge a bit shaken and wondering what lies ahead. I vacillate from a deep appreciation of doctors' abilities to heal to a resentment of the pain their "cures" inflict. Although I knew that Natalie would suffer without the treatment, watching her receive injection after injection as she lies pinned, frightened, and screaming on an x-ray table rips at my soul. It is so depressing to see children in the clinic who have lost their hair and who appear terribly frail. But meeting a five-year-old who survived neuroblastoma after treatment by the same doctors revives my confidence and hope.

Confronting a serious illness in a young child stirs up tremendous emotions in everyone. When strangers inquire about the tumor under her eye (the standard question is, "Who gave her the black eye?") and then discover that she has cancer, they usually are stunned, embarrassed, and incapable of responding. They seem threatened by the awareness that even little babies are prey to cancer, a disease that has become a metaphor for all of our worst fears. I find it difficult to know what to do with their discomfort and sympathy.

I am constantly conflicted over whether to express or suppress what I am feeling. The possibility of a virtual Pandora's box of emotions erupting is both overwhelming and frightening. Some days I'd like not to feel at all; other days I'm truly grateful that I have the capacity for deep emotions.

Conjure up an image of a person strapped to a chair with a time bomb placed on her lap and you will perceive the tension and frustration I experience on a daily basis. In an hour, I go through anxiety, denial, anger, loneliness, and fear. The bomb keeps ticking as I struggle to defuse it. Acknowledging that I don't have the power to remove this threat, and giving up a sense of control over life, has been difficult. I have slowly begun to adjust to the idea that the reality of my life includes death and loss. I had to give up the belief that as long as I was a decent person it was only fair that everything in my life should go smoothly. I had to let God have control.

Coming to grips with my relationship to God has been a difficult task. It is so easy to feel either guilty and accountable for this affliction or angry that a loving God could permit it. I had two choices: bitterness or faith. I chose faith, the belief that there is purpose and meaning here beyond what I presently comprehend. A Bible verse from 2 Timothy has encouraged me: "For God hath not given us the spirit of fear, but of power, and of love, and of a sound mind."

Love is powerful and paradoxical: it binds us to each other and then gives us the capacity to let go. I know Natalie feels loved. That enables me to release her if I must. But loving unselfishly is difficult. I have to enlist the rational me to combat pity, fear, and depression. Self-talk has become an extremely important means of coping. I try to reframe the picture I have of my circumstances, placing each obstacle in a positive framework. Sometimes I don't succeed, and then it is important to allow myself to get depressed and to experience my feelings. I try not to deny myself some sadness when it is appropriate.

I had to learn not to allow my desensitization to the horror of the situation to frighten me. At first I wondered why I answered mechanically when I responded to the inquiries of friends. Now I realize that I couldn't have survived if my emotional temperature had stayed high all the time. What may have appeared callous to others is really an enormous effort to defuse debilitatingly explosive feelings.

It has been difficult but necessary to enlist the support of friends and family. I was accustomed to being the supporter, rarely the supportee. Natalie's illness and the demands of her care have helped me realize that receiving is also a form of loving. Asking for help when it's needed requires courage. It is a way of acknowledging that I am human and that the person giving me support is important.

The significance of my experience resides in paradox. In relinquishing control, I have gained a new kind of power. In accepting death, I have begun to understand life. In being willing to let Natalie go, I have loved her the most that I can.

BRENDA G. STONE is currently completing course work for a Ph.D. in counseling psychology at Texas A & M University. She and her family live in Houston, Texas.

20

Dealing with Death

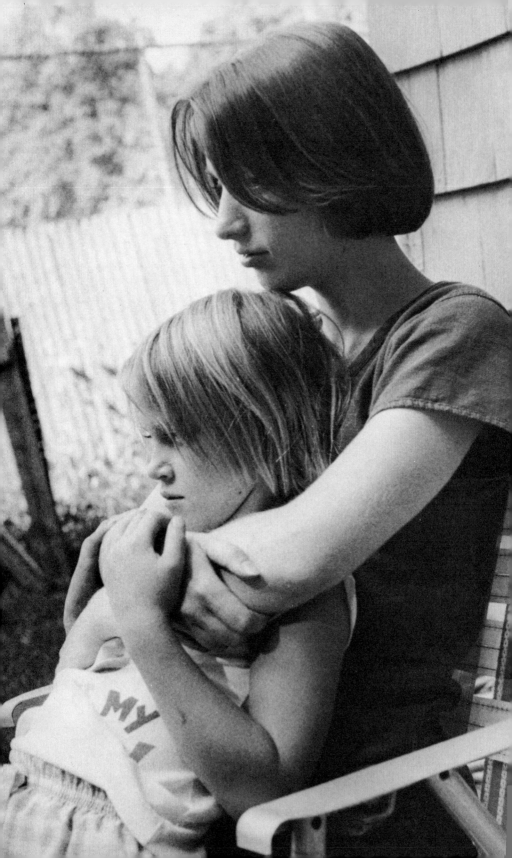

Diary of a Miscarriage

JANE FORSYTH

Miscarriage is perhaps the only phenomenon in which an individual experiences the death of another literally inside her, literally attached to her. Thus the expression "I feel like something in me has died" acquires a special significance. To be so closely attached first to life and then to death brings one's own mortality to consciousness, increasing one's sense of vulnerability and forcing one to confront issues of control, lack of integration, depression, guilt, fear, and anger. My miscarriage involved eight days. This is a record of three of those days.

Day One
I remember Mary Martin saying
Tinkerbell would live if the audience clapped
Hard enough
I stand up in my chair and clap like no tomorrow
Yet she can't hear me
For the audience is filing out
shuffling their feet
hiding wet tissues in the cups of their hands.

Tink's light flickers at fewer intervals
She drops to the floor from a higher perch
Powerless, I watch from my seat
Clapping my prayers to random spirits
(To the deus ex machina no less!)
Clapping my heart out.

I run down the center aisle to the stage
A black pit, cluttered with folding chairs,
Lies between us
No way to reach her
So I clap
Until my hands are red and swollen

One fool clapping, hysterically,
Missing the moment
Dodging the issue.

Tinkerbell is dying, Jane,
Maybe you have time
To hold your hands and cry
Before they lock this place up
For the night.

Day Two

I've been bleeding for over a week now, and I'm literally drained. Clumps of toilet paper have been replaced by more efficient mini-pads — a sign that miscarriage is inevitable. I feel shackled to my bedpost, my toilet, my slippers and waistless clothes. I am in a kind of purgatory: I cannot go forward to a new life; I cannot go back to the time I was filled with a life; I can only stay implanted with the dying or the dead. The blood is brown; it's lost its color. My odor is offensive. I am buried alive — a nightmare out of my childhood realized.

I tried to put an end to the waiting today. I made an appointment with my doctor. The waiting room was empty except for my friend. A door opened, and the nurse beckoned me inside. She knew. She bit her lip and made a sad mime face to tell me she cared. This time there was no weighing in; there were no bad jokes about the monthly urine specimen; just instructions to remove only my underpants. I arranged them on the toilet seat so the blood wouldn't show.

The doctor entered and was gone before I took one breath. But in that moment, he determined through some apparatus akin to a transistor radio that there was no heartbeat pumping within me. He went on to do an internal exam and stated that my uterus was underdeveloped for this stage of my pregnancy. I was still hearing his words about no heartbeat. There was total stillness for a long minute — then a tap on the leg and, "Get dressed and come on in to my office." In a trance, I obeyed.

Although he told me what I knew already, it didn't feel superfluous. His terminology was giving definition and form to my amorphous state. He was labeling and categorizing, Dewey decimal-style, and it felt oddly good to belong to some grouping. His words hit straight and hard; I appreciated them and hated them simultaneously. I only wish he'd have looked at me so I could have cried. But he was hiding while I sat in the middle of his leather chair, staring at his ink blotter and pictures of his children, feeling totally exposed and vulnerable.

I took a breath and asked what options I had if I wished to hasten the miscarriage. He suggested a sonogram to confirm the assumption that the fetus was indeed dead. The ensuing procedure would be a D and C, and would most probably be performed the following day.

Some moments later, I moved to the outer office. The receptionist was talking to me, and I realized she was listing the next steps to take by the way she used her counting finger. I asked her to please write down what she was saying because I was having trouble listening. She mocked my request and laughed. I was angry at her insensitivity, yet I remained mute while she scribbled the instructions on the back of an appointment card.

A wisp of myself passed into the sleeves of my coat and down the hall and front steps and out the door into winter and the parking lot and into the car and home without ever feeling the warmth of my wool coat, the hardness of black asphalt underfoot, the coldness of December, or the motion of the automobile. But I was aware of my friend. I rode home on her caring.

Day Three, Part 1
My husband and I reported to x-ray at exactly nine o'clock. The chief of obstetrics was expecting me; he was expecting a name, one Jane Forsyth, a referral. I could see in his eyes that he had no recollection of our past meeting — no memory of my beautiful black-eyed daughter whom he had helped into this world — no memory of scraping out the remains of a dead fetus from a previous miscarriage. With that realization, I grew small and cold and frightened. My husband gripped my hand tightly. The doctor indicated that he would meet with us in his office afterward to discuss the results of the sonogram. The white-haired Mercury, delivering early morning messages throughout the catacombs of well-buffed floors, disappeared as quickly as he had come. Then came the usher, a sullen spirit with a neatly typed name tag who guided me to a

335

dressing room. I was to shed all my worldly possessions, replacing them with the institution's gray and white sheetwear. I kept on my knee socks, however, blue and green argyles that softly hugged my calves. They weren't going to get all of me. I was aware that my pride and dignity had slipped to my feet — a good place for them to take a stand.

I passed by my husband, who sat cross-legged in the waiting room. We made faces at each other. Neither of us spoke. I carried his look of love and pain down the hall until it fused with my own.

In a dark room full of medical monitors, bleep noises, and mysterious graphs, I lay beneath a large stainless-steel crucifix while it recorded sound waves and miraculously transcribed them into a television picture of my uterus. The screen flickered in my peripheral vision. Patients are not permitted to view themselves, in any way.

Two lab technicians discussed an "interesting case" as they stared routinely at my uterus, checking off what they thought they were observing. I felt that if any one had a right to look at my uterus, it was I. But the way things were set up, it was physically impossible to do that. Angry thoughts stayed within me, never making it to the outside, never given passage by lips now so dry they cracked from no contact. One technician took notice of the amniotic sac and was ready to comment; the other silenced him. I was told to go upstairs to my doctor. My report would follow me. Yet it would arrive before I would.

————————

It was now thirteen-and-one-half weeks from conception. The doctor informed us that our fetus had died in the ninth or tenth week. I noted that this had been a time of ambivalence for us. This was not a statement of guilt but one of respect that perhaps life has a few choices from the very beginning. We were told that the sac had hung on tenaciously while the fetus had all but decomposed. The tissue would need to be suctioned out — a D and C — an abortion procedure. The doctor would administer a local anesthetic in order that I could be a "transient admission" — in at twelve, out by five.

> In at twelve
> Out by five

Nothing in me
Is still alive

He could fit me in that very day. A lunch-break procedure. I had
not planned to stay.

Day Three, Part 2
The struggle continues
Mind and Body
A split integrity
A futile battle
Control marks the spoils for one contestant
Releases the goal of the other
Mind accuses Body: "Deceiver!" "Traitor!" "Sell-Out!"
Body stands unmoved
Discharging only what it needs to

Mind takes a new tack
Playing up, soft-talking
Out and out cajolery
Body stands unmoved
Discharging only what it needs to

Drugs come to "take the edge off"
Mind is lost without the "edge"
So Body sucks in the juice
In a half-assed attempt
To quiet the Mind
Small victory, awareness,
At these times

Body accepts a ride
In a wheeled chariot
Down a green hallway to a room marked "Delivery"
Mind, envisioning a death row journey, balks
Starts formulating arguments
For a stay of execution
Body sits unmoved
Discharging only what it needs to

The table confronts the contestants:

Is it a rack for a pinioned animal?
Or a resting place for a tired woman?

Body, responsible, stops its discharging
Faces Mind
And with compassion
Takes Mind in
In one long, slow, deep breath
Tucking it close to Heart
In the most protected space

And in a pumping rhythm
Orchestrated by Body
Mind chants in a voice
As strong as its captor
"I am my body
I'm larger than the pain"
"I am my body
I'm larger than the pain"
And in the end
When the task at hand was done
Mind and Body were moved
Discharging what they needed to

*After five years in the public schools working as an adolescent and
parent counselor, JANE FORSYTH is currently involved in a full-time
private practice doing individual, group, and family therapy. Jane has been
married eleven years and has two children. She lives in Lexington, Massachusetts.*

Giving Birth to a Child Who Dies

JOAN BRADLEY

It had been a difficult pregnancy. Intermittent bleeding, constant fatigue, and vulnerability to every virus around added up to the danger of miscarriage. I was advised to rest often, but with two small children at home this was almost impossible. The oldest child had just started kindergarten and was having some difficulty adjusting to school. The three-year-old was prone to asthma attacks. Both my daughters needed special care, but I felt incapable of caring for anyone.

We struggled along and then one morning, in my sixth month, labor began. I should have been prepared for the tragedy that was to follow. Very little encouragement was offered by anyone. The volunteer who met me at the emergency room and took me to the maternity floor stated flatly: "You don't look very pregnant. It will be a miracle if they can save your baby." At that point I still believed in miracles.

In the labor room I was alone. Those were the days when the father was an unwelcome presence during childbirth. The nurse examined me from time to time and checked the progress of the labor. I had been given medication that was supposed to stop the contractions, but it didn't work. I heard the nurse telephoning the doctor: "Contractions regular. Dilation five centimeters." By early evening I was in the delivery room.

She was born quickly, this tiny little girl. Something like a veil covered her face. "It's the membranes from the amniotic sac," the doctor explained, "the caul of old wives' tales. It is supposed to mean a special child, a prophetic child." She weighed twenty-four ounces and measured fourteen inches long. Her cry was a gasp for air. I watched the nurse cradle my daughter who was wrapped in a warm blanket, and baptize her as I had requested. "Her name is Elizabeth Ann," I said. The doctor looked up and counseled quietly, "Don't hope, please, don't hope. She is much too small to survive." I reached out and touched her as she was carried past me. So small, so terribly fragile, she kept her eyes shut tightly and waved her tiny fists in the air as she struggled for breath in this strange new world.

The team from the neonatal intensive care unit was waiting at the door. She was placed in an incubator and taken away. All the equipment and expertise of modern medicine were being utilized to keep this frail being alive. I still believed in miracles.

My husband joined me briefly in the recovery room. He was smiling and telling me not to worry. He hadn't seen our baby but felt certain that everything would be all right. I tried to match his optimism but was too exhausted physically to share his enthusiasm. My body was numb from the exertion of bringing this child into the world and tense with the anxiety of wondering what would happen to her. We made plans concerning what we needed to purchase and make ready at home for this early arrival. My husband left to make phone calls and promised to be right back.

When he returned the pediatrician was with him. "I can't detect a heartbeat," the doctor said, "and her lungs will not function. I'm sorry. We did what we could." I nodded, not trusting myself to speak, and turned to my husband; his face was devastated.

The doctor continued: "She has to be buried. It's a state law. Do you know of a funeral home you could notify? They will take care of things." My husband said he would make arrangements. Suddenly I felt chilled; I began to tremble. The nurse immediately gave me a shot of something that brought an end to the horrible reality.

———————

The following morning the real nightmare began. There was a constriction in my throat, and I could manage neither breakfast nor conversation with the chaplain who came to visit. He was followed by a woman from the hospital records department who needed information for two legal certificates: one for birth and one for death. I was deeply distressed, but it had to be done.

My husband called to tell me about the funeral arrangements. The baby would be buried on the following day with a simple graveside service. Although it could have been arranged, I didn't want to be there.

The doctor arrived before noon. "It's probably for the best," he said sympathetically. "Premature birth, immature lungs, she

340

might have been a vegetable." I stared at him numbly and thought, She was *my* vegetable; she was *my* baby.

———————

When I returned home my children responded with pleasure at seeing me again. They wanted to know if I would feel better now and not be sick all the time. I fervently hoped so. The death of their infant sister meant very little to them.

Friends and neighbors came by to see me and attempted words of comfort. None of their comments made sense to me. "You are still young enough to have more babies. You can replace this one." But this child could never be replaced. She was uniquely herself. She would never be a part of my life. I had been denied the chance to mother her, to hold her, to love her.

"You have two fine children. You should be grateful for what you have." I wasn't feeling grateful to anyone for anything. I was feeling a terrible sense of emptiness and failure. This was compounded by normal postpartum fatigue and hormonal changes.

"She didn't live long enough for you to really get to know her" was a frequent comment. But she was known to me. The only life that baby knew was in my body. I felt her movements, heard her heartbeat. For six months we were involved in a deeply personal relationship. Seeing her born, hearing her cry, and touching her were extremely intimate events.

"Just keep busy and get on with things. You'll recover quickly since you can sleep at night." But I didn't sleep at night. The sound of a baby's cry would reach me although no baby was there. Night after night, while my family slept, I would sit in the rocking chair wishing the baby were with me. The sleeplessness persisted for several weeks.

My days continued. In a stupor, I cared for my children, household chores, and other monotonous activities; but my mind was elsewhere. I cried a lot. I wanted to talk about the baby, but most people were uncomfortable with the subject. Only with my husband and my children could I work through the grief.

Eventually the wounds healed both physically and emotionally, but the scar remains. We still talk about Elizabeth Ann, particularly on her birthday. My daughters question me: "How old

341

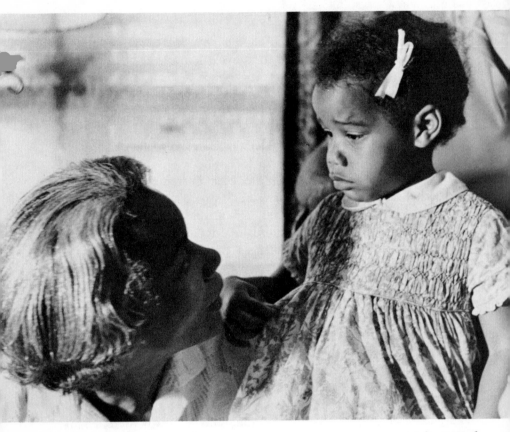

Julie O'Neil

would she be now? Would she be in school? What grade? Would she look like me?" I visit her grave and remember this tiny person who touched me so briefly and so deeply.

I have accepted her death. And yet last spring, when I again became pregnant, my twelve-year-old daughter reported a strange dream in which a little girl kept calling for Mommy. The dream was so vivid that my daughter awoke to look for the child. We hadn't told the children about my pregnancy and when we finally did announce that a new baby was on the way, my daughter remembered her dream. Her interpretation was, "It is Elizabeth Ann and she wants us to know everything will be all right this time." And everything was all right this time.

JOAN BRADLEY and her family are residents of the Los Angeles area. At thirty-nine, she entered college part-time and, despite the arrival of a new baby, is continuing her education.

"Something Must Have Gone Wrong"
FRANCOISE E. THEISE

It was my first pregnancy. I was the center of attention. I was full of energy. I was glowing. I was at the end of my thirty-sixth week, and the baby's room was almost ready to receive her (somehow I knew it would be a girl). Some superstitious friends made me feel that we had prepared the room too early, but it didn't worry me.

After a busy day, I was finally relaxing and realized that I hadn't felt the baby move all day. I had read that toward the end of pregnancy babies get comfortable and do not move as much. However, I was concerned and decided to call my doctor first thing in the morning if I still had not felt her moving.

Without telling anyone, I went to my doctor's office that next morning. "We will pick up the heartbeat on our monitor, and you will feel better," he reassured me. But he couldn't hear anything. I felt chills and hot rushes at the same time. He was avoiding my eyes and said, "It doesn't look too good, but we'll send you to the hospital where they can sometimes do better than we can with a fetal monitor. Don't get your hopes up too high."

Hope? I knew my baby was dead. I knew there was no hope; my body told me that there was no life inside it.

I couldn't believe it was happening to me — a normal, healthy, twenty-seven-year-old woman. Susan, the nurse, was holding my hand. I wanted her to hold me tighter but couldn't ask. I couldn't shed a tear. We took a cab to the hospital after calling my husband and leaving a message for him to meet me there, revealing nothing else.

During the cab ride, Susan didn't talk. It was just as well because I wouldn't have heard her. A thousand thoughts were going through my mind at the same time: What happened? What did I do? Is it because I played tennis until my seventh month? Oh, how is Jay going to react? The baby's room is all set. Who will have to take it apart? Why us? I took such good care of myself, and all my checkups were fine. I never took any medicine. Something is wrong with my body. I am not as healthy as I thought. My friends shouldn't have given me a baby shower so soon. I would like my mother to be near me now. I remember clearly that all these thoughts were coming at me in no special order, and I had barely thought of the baby and how it was going to be delivered.

At the hospital I was sitting in the registration office waiting to be taken to the labor floor when someone behind a desk started asking me questions, such as whether I wanted pictures to be taken of my baby; or, if it were a boy, would he be circumcised in the hospital. It was horrible. Fortunately Susan came to my rescue. I felt too panicked to talk to anyone, especially to strangers.

Entering the labor room, I felt cheated. I remembered our visit to this floor during one of the prenatal classes. I had been dreaming of the day I would come back with Jay and my suitcase, ready to master all the contractions. I had practiced my breathing exercises and read every book on pregnancy and delivery that I could find. I felt like a student who had flunked her exams.

The next thing I knew I was in a bed with electrodes all over me. They were going to try to see the baby's heartbeat transferred on the graph.

Why did they have to do this? I knew beyond a doubt that my baby was dead. I felt empty and terribly tired. I didn't stop them because it was a way for everyone to show me that there was no fetal heartbeat on the graph: they couldn't say it to me; it had to be seen.

Still I couldn't cry. Susan assured me it was okay, that crying would be good for me. But I was with strangers and couldn't let go. I needed a friend or a relative who knew me as the happy, healthy expectant mother and therefore understood the shock I was experiencing.

Finally Jay arrived. I saw that he must have gone home to change; he was carrying his camera. Obviously he had thought he was being called for an early delivery. The nurse had caught him outside the door and explained the situation to him. I think I finally burst into tears because I knew how he felt at that moment. He was desperately trying to hide his sadness, his deep disappointment. He smiled and we held each other tightly. I could have cried a long time.

At that point everybody had finally agreed that the baby was not alive. The doctor gave me a choice that at first left me speechless: I could either be induced or carry the baby until I went into normal labor. At the time I hadn't heard of women who had had to carry their dead baby until term, so it sounded like a cruel thing to propose as an option. Now I understand that the doctors were trying to spare me intense physical pain and risks. Almost instantly, and with anger, I said, "I will not leave this hospital until you deliver my baby." I didn't even ask Jay what he thought. I desperately wanted to be freed of my baby who was no longer moving and was no longer making my body feel vibrant, as it had for the past eight months. I was very drained, very tired. I wanted to be able to start from zero by taking the baby out of my body. That same big, round body I had loved and fondled with such warmth and pride now made me cry. I wanted to see it flat again.

The labor was extremely painful. There was almost no rest period between contractions, and at times it seemed my body was literally being thrown off the bed. I don't think I'll ever be able to explain the sensation clearly. They would not give me any pain medication because it would have slowed down the whole process. And I agreed; I wanted it to be over as soon as possible.

I was in labor all day. Susan returned from work to be near me. My doctor, however, turned me over to his associate just as I was at the peak of my labor and close to delivery. It angered me to be with a stranger at that traumatic time.

Finally they wheeled me into the delivery room. So far everything I had read about the various phases of labor was true, except that there was nothing exciting to look forward to at the end of the arduous road. I had asked to be under general anesthesia. I didn't want to know my baby. I didn't want to see it all formed, as a real person. Yet when no one said anything about the baby, I asked, "What was it? How big?" My husband answered that it was a little girl, four-and-a-half pounds. I knew it, I said. For the first time I cried for my little girl. I wanted that baby to be in our arms with her heart beating strongly. Oh! Did I miss her!

What happened? They don't know. The cord was not around the neck. They didn't find any antibodies that might have been caused by my Rh negative blood type. They would have to do an autopsy. This was the beginning of a miserable period — not knowing what went wrong. I delivered a perfect little baby girl, but her heart was not beating, and nobody knew why.

Back in my room, I felt empty, hating the flat stomach that I had longed for.

———————

Leaving the hospital empty-handed was devastating. I couldn't look at pregnant women; I envied them, and they instantly drew tears out of me. I was frightened to see people, maybe embarrassed. The only thing I could say to my in-laws and my husband was, "I am sorry." I felt that I had disappointed them all, that I had somehow failed. The only person I didn't feel like apologizing to was my mother. She came right away from France and was waiting for me. She had arranged fresh flowers everywhere. She was feeling as sad as I that this tragedy was happening to her own child.

I needed my husband near me, but I especially needed my mother. She was another woman, and she loved me. With her I could cry and cry without restraint. And I did a lot of that, on and off. My moods would fluctuate radically in the same day — up one minute, down the next.

I peeked into what was going to be our baby's room. It was empty. My mother-in-law had called the store, and they had picked up everything. Since then, we never used that room for anything else; I believed that a baby would be in it some day. Was that our way of grieving?

At times, I was strangely optimistic. Since it was a "freak accident," the chances of its recurrence were almost nil. We liked thinking that it was fate. Perhaps even if they had delivered the baby earlier, something chemically wrong would have developed later on.

I desperately wanted to be pregnant again, but the doctor advised me to wait until my body had time to recover, about four months. It seemed like a period of years.

My husband, I believe, had the toughest role. He had been with me through the whole labor; he had sobbed into the nurse's arms so that he could keep a smile for me, dealt with signing papers authorizing the hospital to take care of the autopsy and the burial, and then he went right back to work. He always tried to come home early, not to find comfort, but to give me comfort and hold me while I cried. He put all his energy into helping me pull out of my depression and get strong again, especially after my mother left and we were forced to face our terrible sadness alone. It is only then that it caught up with him, and he also cried bitterly.

At that time I felt capable of putting all my energies into consoling him. Although we didn't need that kind of test, our tragedy definitely brought us closer together. We learned a great deal about each other. We also feel that a weak relationship would not have survived such trying times. We cried together and talked and talked, but our difficult times were not over yet: we both wanted to be pregnant so badly that we tried too hard, and "making love" took on a completely different role. It was for business, not pleasure. No matter how hard we tried not to, pregnancy was all we discussed.

We even stopped seeing certain friends who had been expecting at the same time as we were and had delivered normal, beautiful babies. They understood and were patient. When we do see them, even now, we can't help looking at the children and thinking, Our child would have been the same age. What would she have been like?

I would inevitably bump into people who had last seen me when I was pregnant. They asked the obvious question, "So what did you have?" They assumed that I had been pregnant and then had delivered a healthy baby. I couldn't say I had a miscarriage; it was more than that. And I couldn't say that the baby died; that word didn't come out. I answered, "I lost the baby." What a strange expression! Fortunately no one asked any further questions; they didn't know what to say either. Since then, I have consciously waited for couples to announce the birth of a baby before I ask any questions.

———

We now have two healthy, wonderful children, but we shall never forget our first baby; she is part of us. Every year in May we feel terribly sad. We will always wonder what went wrong, and why us?

Raised and educated in France, FRANCOISE E. THEISE came to this country on an exchange teaching program. She returned to work after the death of her child. "It helped me to focus on other people and push aside, for part of the day, my strong desire to become pregnant again."

21

*Dealing
with the Future*

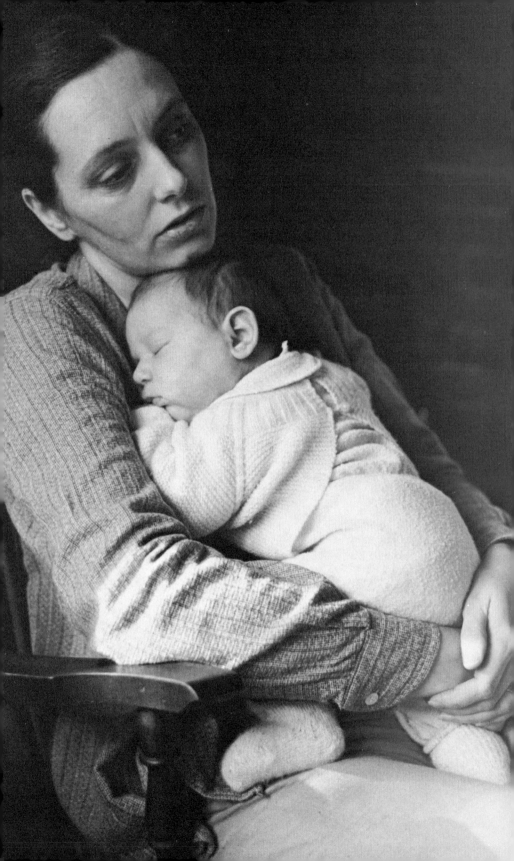

Plague

KINERETH GENSLER

The locusts are swarming inside our children

They have waited us out, dormant
in their inexorable cycle
while we gave TLC & vaccines
against diphtheria, whooping cough, scarlet fever
against smallpox & poliomyelitis

They waited, patient as intelligence agents
till the children's teeth
were straightened and their acne
cleared and their eyes
adjusted to contact lenses
Then they swarmed

This is the year of their swarming

the air is black
the windows of our small town
are blurred we can barely see
for the black cloud eating its way
through our children

one by motorcycle
one by drowning
one by overdose
one by trainwheels
one by stabbing
one with her long hair shining
alone in a barn, yesterday

Plague is upon us, contagion
death of the first-born
and of the second-born

we are helpless to say goodbye, Sally
Michael, Danny, Karen, Kirk, Ann

We are helpless to help each other

On Despair, Hope, and Motherhood

ELEANOR MAHAR DEEGAN

For me, the decision to have a baby was a leap of faith. I had been a handicapped child, having inherited a complicated congenital skeletal deformity from my father. My mother had gone through three miscarriages and a stillbirth before successfully giving birth to me: and she then went through the ordeal of mothering a severely handicapped child who spent most of her first six years in and out of the hospital. I think that it was more difficult for her than for me, since she felt guilty and empathized with my pain and trauma perhaps more than she should have. In those days, there hadn't been much in the way of counseling for parents of special-needs children, and hers had been a lonely struggle.

Having my baby was a calculated risk. There was a fifty-fifty chance that the child would be affected by the mutant gene. Within that fifty-fifty chance, there was a wide range of possible involvement, from so severe that I would spontaneously abort, to so minor that the deformity would not be apparent.

From the moment my pregnancy was confirmed I was, to say the least, cautious. I wanted a child. I was over thirty; the time was now. Pregnancy and childbirth are always a risk, I told myself, and went on to make secret pacts with God, bargaining shamelessly for my child. Let me have this baby and I will do everything right. I promised to be the best mother ever. For nine months I held my existential breath, praying and pleading and promising perfection, reading everything I could, listening to everyone, taking the best possible care of myself and the little creature who grew inside of me.

My daughter was born in September of 1976. She was delivered by Caesarean section, and when I awoke in the recovery room, my husband, Thomas, was there with me. "It's a girl," he said softly, "seven pounds, six ounces, and she's perfect." I remember the overwhelming surge of relief, the tears welling up. "You're sure they got the right baby?"

He was sure.

When we brought her home five days later, I was overjoyed, depleted, exhausted, and thankful. We had defied the odds — Thomas, Deidre, and I — and we had won. We were blessed. She was hard won and precious, and we would do everything in our power to repay the gods.

This child would have the best of everything. Thomas and I had gone through a lot to get where we were that day, had worked hard to overcome a plethora of personal problems in our six years of marriage to become who we were: two reasonably sane, reasonably healthy, loving human beings. It had taken much courage and not a little faith and we were, it is safe to say, proud of ourselves. Finally the ordeal was over. No more sleepless nights of anxiety, no more unknown possibilities. The world was safe again. I had visions of Thomas, the baby, and I growing together in loving harmony and struggle (I had no illusions about life being easy). Deidre would grow to adulthood in the safe harbor of our love, much as she had grown to birth in the warmth of my womb. Then she would leave us, of course, to be born as an adult in her own life, and Thomas and I would grow old and wise together. It was a vision born of the heady sense of victory.

Over the next two weeks, I slept and ate and fed and cuddled and cried soft tears of wonder. I was totally involved with my baby. I was reading Spock religiously (Deidre was colicky), calling people to share our joy, starting a baby book, doing all the things I wanted to do and all the things I thought I should do. I watched my diet to make sure that there would be nothing upsetting in my milk, used corn starch instead of talcum powder on her little bum, and spent enormous amounts of time stroking her, talking to her, making her

353

feel safe. When the real world came crashing into our small, safe one, I wasn't prepared and I was nearly devastated.

———————

It happened on a rainy autumn evening. I was sitting in the living room, nursing Deidre, listening to the soft rain outside, half watching the news, half lost in the reverie of nursing. Tom was in the kitchen fixing supper. Everything was warm, cozy, safe. The real world intruded through the voice of the six o'clock newscaster. I was looking at Deidre, at her intense little face, feeling her soft, warm mouth on my breast, adjusting the shawl that was slipping off my shoulders, when I heard that the soft autumn rain that was falling so gently, so reassuringly outside the window was no ordinary rain. This rain, in the month of my daughter's birth, in the days of our golden possibility, was dangerous, radioactive, potentially deadly rain that was falling from a huge killer cloud that had made its way to us from halfway around the world: a birthday present from the People's Republic of China. Best to stay inside, the newscaster was saying. Best to drink bottled water. Best to . . . best to . . .

I remember sitting very still. I remember the chill down my spine and the sudden sour taste of panic in my mouth. I remember the tears clouding my vision and sliding slowly down my face as I moved Deidre gently to my shoulder. I tried not to sob, not to move in a manner that would be disruptive to my baby. The elation of the last two weeks evaporated like illusion in the damp evening air.

Take Deidre, run. Run hard, run fast. Run away. Where? Run where? My stomach was churning, my heart pounding. There wasn't, I knew deep in my mother's heart, anywhere to go. It wasn't fair. We had worked so hard, fought so well. She was fine and normal and we were all prepared and now this. There could be no bargaining with God this time, no deal I could strike to protect her from this. I felt desperate, totally helpless.

Two years later, in the wake of the accident at Three Mile Island, I heard a mother from Harrisburg say essentially the same thing: the reality of possible accidents at your local power plants made a mockery of motherhood. You do everything right, she said, you get them their shots and you make them brush their teeth and you read all the books, and then this happens.

But in the fall of 1976, Three Mile Island and the consciousness it raised were still two-and-a-half years away. The nuclear rain that terrorized my new mother's heart opened floodgates of feelings I had never connected with motherhood. Suddenly my decision to have Deidre and my vision of our future as a family seemed selfish and naive. Guilt sat squarely on my shoulder and whispered in my ear. Had I brought my beautiful little girl into the world only to have her poisoned slowly by radiation, or killed instantly by nuclear holocaust? What could I do to make it safe for her, in the face of such monstrous possibilities?

So began the winter of my despair. I read the newspapers compulsively, obsessively poring over each page, as if by overdosing on horror I could make it magically disappear. In despair, I began to understand for the first time how it was that a mother could kill herself, putting her head in the gas oven after setting out breakfast for her babies, as Sylvia Plath had done. Why not, guilt whispered, what else can you do?

At this point I wasn't at all sure I was sane. Many a long cold winter's night I lay awake, Thomas asleep beside me, Deidre bundled in her bassinet, trying to escape the visions of horror, the free-floating fear that wouldn't leave me in peace. There didn't seem to be anywhere to turn for help. Then I would doubt my sanity; maybe it wasn't the world; maybe *I* was the problem. Maybe the fears and the panic were just sublimated anxieties over being a mother that I couldn't admit to myself. Maybe it was all a case of postpartum depression and raging hormonal imbalances.

I was too confused, too frightened, and all too well convinced of my own capacity for neurosis to share my feelings with anyone. The tremendous guilt I was feeling grew stronger, feeding on my loneliness. Not only had I brought my child into what I now saw as a doomed world, but I was depressed all the time as well. I felt as if I were on a slick slide, grabbing at the railings to keep from plummeting out of control into the unknown. Each morning I would resolve anew not to feel what I was feeling. Each day I would work hard at pretending I wasn't insane, begging my daughter's forgiveness silently in my heart, treating her with the tenderness one reserves for the doomed.

Somewhere in the middle of that awful lonely winter, I had a dream that began my resurrection. It was so vivid that it woke me.

In the dream, I was standing in an alley waiting to meet my mother. (In reality, my mother has been dead for seven years.) She joined me in the alley and asked me to walk with her for awhile, since she had been given special leave to talk with me. She was dressed shabbily, but she had about her an aura of loving urgency, and I listened carefully to what she said. She told me that the future was bleak, bleaker than anything she had lived through, and she had lived through two world wars and the depression. She told me that there was no way out. She told me that I had to be strong, as strong as I had been as a child when I had had to learn to walk anew after each operation. She told me that she loved me.

I woke up from that dream lonely and shivering, wanting to go with her, wanting her to come back, but feeling somehow saner and safer. She was right and I knew it. Because of Deidre, the world, too, was my responsibility. Somehow, somewhere I had to find the strength to fight for it and to fight for her and for all of the children everywhere.

The help I needed in pointing the way came to me in the form of the women's movement. Adrienne Rich's book *Of Woman Born* was published that winter, and following some serendipitous instinct, I read it greedily. It didn't make everything better; it didn't make the horror go away. If anything, it deepened the horror, delving as it does into the dark, hidden realities of motherhood as it exists within the confines of the patriarchy. What it did do was confirm my sanity and the appropriateness of my responses. And it made me realize that I was not alone. By breaking the silence, it helped me to find my tongue.

I began to see that as a mother I was hostage to the future of a world dominated by the patriarchal value system of competition and mastery, a system which was now and had always been in dangerous opposition to the process of mothering. The present was only the terminal stage, the final culmination of centuries. The scope of the technology was what was new, nothing else. The guns had always been aimed at us, the women and the children and the gentle men; it was just that now they were bigger than ever, final in capabilities.

As my knowledge of the depth of what it was I was fighting increased, as I learned how entrenched and powerful the patriarchy really was, controlling as it does no less than the whole world, I

Pat Wells

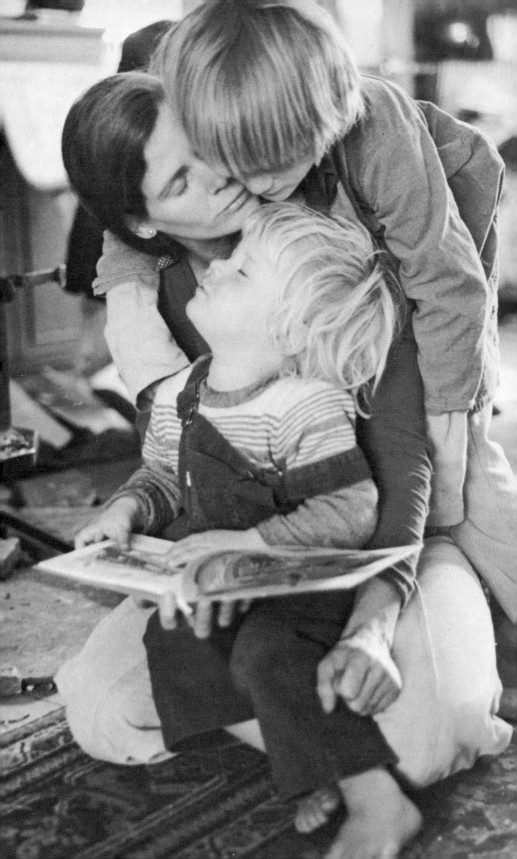

became more convinced that there was much to fear. But understanding evaporated my guilt and gave me hope, no matter how tenuous. And hope spurred me to action. I began, with trepidation, to talk about what I was feeling. Much to my relief, I found out I wasn't alone among the women I knew. Many of them had shared my feelings of terror and loneliness when the full reality of the future hit them after they had given birth to their children. Talking about it opened repressed feelings in them as well as in me, not the least of which was anger. I discovered that rage is a wonderful antidote to despair.

In the three-and-a-half years since that Chinese cloud, many things have happened in the world which make our responsibilities even more overwhelming. It is a dazzling leap of faith to mother in a world that may already be dying.

———————

As Deidre grows and I watch her unfolding like a flower in the morning sun, I know I can do nothing else. I have come to see political action as a part of mothering, as necessary and as important as finding shoes that fit and as telling nighttime stories. Right now, I am putting most of my energies into the antinuclear movement because I see the possibility of nuclear annihilation as the most urgent threat to my daughter's well-being. But I also put energy into more strictly feminist activities because I know, as a woman and the mother of a girl, that making the world safe for her involves more than keeping it from being blown up.

I still have sleepless nights, still sink into despair. But I am no longer alone and I no longer feel totally helpless. I can live with myself and I can live with my daughter, even with the nuclear sword hanging over our heads. I can even find cause to celebrate. After all, together we might save the world.

ELEANOR MAHAR DEEGAN of Cambridge, Massachusetts, has been married for nine years. "My daughter is three years old now and used to her mother's political activities. All in all, despite everything in this crazy world, I am glad that I chose to have her."

Notes on Contributing Poets and Photographers

Notes on Contributing Poets

CAROL HOFFMAN DeCANIO is a thirty-seven-year-old published poet who lives in Santa Barbara, California, with her husband and their two sons.

KINERETH GENSLER, mother of three grown children, teaches poetry writing in the Radcliffe Seminars. Her book of poems, *Without Roof*, will be published by Alice James Books in the spring of 1981. She is a resident of Belmont, Massachusetts.

CAROL KORT is co-editor of this book. Her poems have appeared in *Sojourner, Gnosis*, and the *Tufts Literary Review*.

SUSAN MacDONALD was born and educated in London and now lives in Menlo Park, California, with her two children and her husband. She has published two books, *Dangerous as Daughters* and *A Smart Dithyramb*.

MURIEL RUKEYSER (1913–1980) was a New York City poet, lecturer, teacher, and mother. In addition to five volumes of prose and a number of children's books, she published more than a dozen volumes of poetry. Her work has been translated into ten languages, and her awards included a Guggenheim Fellowship and the National Institute Award.

Notes on Contributing Photographers

JOAN ALBERT is a single parent who generally photographs families. She teaches photography at Project Art Center in Cambridge, Massachusetts.

BETH ANSELL, a mother of two children, lives in Newton, Massachusetts. She was an elementary school teacher in Virginia and has worked as a photographer for a weekly city newspaper, as well as doing freelance work.

BIRGIT BLYTH is a freelance photographer who loves portrait photography because of her fascination with people. A mother of two, she is currently involved in various group shows.

BONNIE BURT helped edit the photography in this book. She is a freelance photographer and psychotherapist living in Cambridge, Massachusetts. Her work has appeared in several college and university publications. Recently she published *At 35*, a limited edition of her work. She is a godmother.

ETHEL DIAMOND, of Fanwood, New Jersey, attended New York University Law School. She has two children and is a self-taught photographer who has been involved in several group shows. Her work has been published in books and magazines such as *Ms.* and *American Photographer*.

"Mother and Child" is a soft-sculpture doll created by LOIS SCHKLAR, a craftswoman whose dolls have been exhibited widely in galleries in Toronto and other parts of Canada. The "Mother and Child" doll is in the collection of Shirley Morris. (Photograph by BRUCE HOGG.)

GAIL LEBOFF studied art in New York City, where she lives, and is currently a photographer. She has exhibited in several galleries, and her photographs have been published.

DANIEL E. LITTLE teaches philosophy at Colgate University. He is the father of Joshua and the husband of Ronnie Friedland.

MARY ANN LYNCH, a Greenfield Center, New York, resident, is a mother of two children. She is editor and publisher of *Combinations: A Journal of Photography*. She has also taught photography and has exhibited her own work throughout the United States.

PEGGY McMAHON is a freelance photographer from Cambridge, Massachusetts. Her photographs have appeared frequently in publications such as the Boston *Phoenix* and *The Village Voice*.

ALICE MOULTON of Concord, Massachusetts, is a freelance photographer working on photographing the elderly in Concord in conjunction with a larger, oral-history project.

JULIE O'NEIL was the photographer for a book about children entitled *Seed Time*. She has taught photography and freelanced for industrial and educational institutions. She is currently involved in capturing the way animals and humans relate and interact.

MELISSA SHOOK is a photographer, writer, and teacher. She has taught photography and self-expression at M.I.T., and her articles have appeared in *Camera 35* and *Photograph*. Portfolios of her photographs have appeared in *Creative Camera* and in the Time-Life book series.

ELLEN SHUB is a Boston-based freelance photographer. Her pictures have appeared in national magazines and books. She is especially interested in documenting political and social issues.

ROBERT BECK STUHLMANN is an Episcopal minister who lives in Jamaica Plain, Massachusetts. He is the father of Christopher — a special-needs child about whom an essay appears in this book.

MARGARET THOMPSON has taken pictures since her childhood days in rural Pennsylvania. Her current, major ongoing projects include photographing American adolescents and northern Kenyan nomads.

PAT WELLS, who lives in Somerville, Massachusetts, taught herself photography. She takes pictures "for love and pleasure."